SpringerBriefs in Statistics

JSS Research Series in Statistics

Editors-in-chief

Naoto Kunitomo
Akimichi Takemura

Series editors

Genshiro Kitagawa
Tomoyuki Higuchi
Nakahiro Yoshida
Yutaka Kano
Toshimitsu Hamasaki
Shigeyuki Matsui
Manabu Iwasaki

The current research of statistics in Japan has expanded in several directions in line with recent trends in academic activities in the area of statistics and statistical sciences over the globe. The core of these research activities in statistics in Japan has been the Japan Statistical Society (JSS). This society, the oldest and largest academic organization for statistics in Japan, was founded in 1931 by a handful of pioneer statisticians and economists and now has a history of about 80 years. Many distinguished scholars have been members, including the influential statistician Hirotugu Akaike, who was a past president of JSS, and the notable mathematician Kiyosi Itô, who was an earlier member of the Institute of Statistical Mathematics (ISM), which has been a closely related organization since the establishment of ISM. The society has two academic journals: the Journal of the Japan Statistical Society (English Series) and the Journal of the Japan Statistical Society (Japanese Series). The membership of JSS consists of researchers, teachers, and professional statisticians in many different fields including mathematics, statistics, engineering, medical sciences, government statistics, economics, business, psychology, education, and many other natural, biological, and social sciences.

The JSS Series of Statistics aims to publish recent results of current research activities in the areas of statistics and statistical sciences in Japan that otherwise would not be available in English; they are complementary to the two JSS academic journals, both English and Japanese. Because the scope of a research paper in academic journals inevitably has become narrowly focused and condensed in recent years, this series is intended to fill the gap between academic research activities and the form of a single academic paper.

The series will be of great interest to a wide audience of researchers, teachers, professional statisticians, and graduate students in many countries who are interested in statistics and statistical sciences, in statistical theory, and in various areas of statistical applications.

More information about this series at http://www.springer.com/series/13497

Toshimitsu Hamasaki · Koko Asakura
Scott R. Evans · Toshimitsu Ochiai

Group-Sequential Clinical Trials with Multiple Co-Objectives

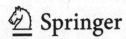

Toshimitsu Hamasaki
Department of Data Science
National Cerebral and Cardiovascular Center
Suita, Osaka
Japan

Koko Asakura
Department of Data Science
National Cerebral and Cardiovascular Center
Suita, Osaka
Japan

Scott R. Evans
Department of Biostatistics and the Center
 for Biostatistics in AIDS Research
Harvard T.H. Chan School of Public Health
Boston, MA
USA

Toshimitsu Ochiai
Biostatistics Department
Shionogi & Co., Ltd.,
Osaka
Japan

ISSN 2191-544X   ISSN 2191-5458   (electronic)
SpringerBriefs in Statistics
ISSN 2364-0057   ISSN 2364-0065   (electronic)
JSS Research Series in Statistics
ISBN 978-4-431-55898-9   ISBN 978-4-431-55900-9   (eBook)
DOI 10.1007/978-4-431-55900-9

Library of Congress Control Number: 2016936577

Printed on acid-free paper

This Springer imprint is published by Springer Nature
The registered company is Springer Japan KK

Contents

Abbreviations

AAD	Antibiotic-Associated Diarrhoea
ADAS-Cog	The Alzheimer Disease Assessment Scale Cognitive Subscale
ADCS-ADL	The Alzheimer Disease Cooperative Study Activities of Daily Living
AON	Average Observation Number
AS	Assay Sensitivity
ASN	Average Sample Number
CDD	C *difficile* diarrhoea
CDF	Cumulative Distribution Function
CHMP	Committee for Medicinal Products for Human Use
CHW	Cui-Hung-Wang
CP	Conditional Power
CPMP	Committee for Proprietary Medical Products
FDA	Food and Drug Administration
IBS	Irritable Bowel Syndrome
ICH	The International Conference on Harmonisation of Technical Requirements for Registration of Pharmaceuticals for Human Use
ITT	Intent-to-Treat
MSS	Maximum Sample Size
NI	Non-inferiority
OF	O'Brien-Fleming
PC	Pocock
PMDA	Pharmaceuticals and Medical Devices Agency
PPS	Per Protocol Set
UPDRS	The Unified Parkinson's Disease Rating Scale

Chapter 1
Introduction

Abstract In this chapter, we provide an overview of several emerging statistical challenges in recent clinical trials. These include multiple endpoints, non-inferiority designs, and adaptive designs.

Keywords Modern adaptive designs · Group-sequential designs · Multiple endpoints · Non-inferiority designs

1.1 Emerging Statistical Issues in Clinical Trials

Clinical trials are the most reliable and well-accepted scientific methods for evaluating the efficacy, safety, and effectiveness of investigational medical products. Clinical trials eliminate or reduce many biases and confounding that plague observational studies through the use of tools such as prospective observation, randomization, blinding, use of control groups, and the intent-to-treat (ITT) principle, to isolate the effect of an intervention and establish cause and effect (Mosteller 1981; Evans and Ting 2015). However, clinical trials can be extremely expensive and resource intensive as they often require the enrollment of large numbers of participants and the collection of massive amounts of data. The high costs of clinical trials have contributed to stagnation in medical product development. The costs are barriers to innovation that might offer patients rapid access to new medical products (Food and Drug Administration, FDA 2006).

To evaluate the most appropriate interventions for future patients, clinical trials are usually conducted to assess whether an improvement of a patient's disease status could be observed with the use of a new intervention, whether adverse reactions are caused by a new intervention, and how a new intervention could physiologically work. Despite clinical trials, considerable uncertainty regarding the safety and effectiveness of medical products often remains. The two major causes are the dearth of knowledge and evaluative tools for exploring pharmacological mechanisms (either of benefit or risk) and the limited ability of clinical trials to address more than a few questions within a single trial (FDA 2006).

T. Hamasaki et al., *Group-Sequential Clinical Trials with Multiple Co-Objectives*,
JSS Research Series in Statistics, DOI 10.1007/978-4-431-55900-9_1

There is demand for new approaches for developing medical products more quickly and more cost effectively. Several statistical challenging areas have emerged in pursuit of more effective and efficient development. These include multiple endpoints, non-inferiority designs, adaptive designs, targeted subgroup and enrichment designs, and multi-regional clinical trial designs. This book focuses on two of these challenges, clinical trials with multiple endpoints and non-inferiority clinical trials, but discusses these within the framework of group-sequential designs.

1.1.1 Multiple Co-primary Endpoints

In clinical trials, most commonly, a single outcome is selected as a primary endpoint and then used as the basis for the trial design including sample size determination, interim data monitoring, final analyses, and reporting and publication of results. However, many recent clinical trials have utilized more than one primary endpoint as co-primary. "Co-primary" means that a trial is designed to evaluate whether a test intervention has an effect on *all* of the primary endpoints. Failure to demonstrate an effect on any single endpoint implies that the beneficial effect to the control intervention cannot be concluded. The rationale for this is that the use of a single endpoint may not provide a comprehensive picture of the intervention's multidimensional effects.

Regulators have issued guidelines recommending multiple co-primary endpoints in specific disease areas including acute heart failure (Committee for Medicinal Products for Human Use, CHMP 2012a), Alzheimer's disease (CHMP 2008; FDA 2013), diabetes mellitus (CHMP 2012b), Duchenne and Becker muscular dystrophy (CHMP 2013a), and irritable bowel syndrome (IBS) (FDA 2012; CHMP 2013b). For example, CHMP (2008) and FDA (2013) recommend a co-primary endpoint approach using cognitive and functional or global endpoints to evaluate symptomatic improvement of dementia associated with Alzheimer's disease, indicating that primary endpoints should be stipulated reflecting the cognitive and functional components. In the design of clinical trials evaluating treatments in patients affected by IBS, the FDA recommends the use of two co-primary endpoints for assessing IBS signs and symptoms: (1) pain intensity and stool frequency of IBS with constipation (IBS-C) and (2) pain intensity and stool consistency of IBS with diarrhea (IBS-D) (FDA 2012). CHMP (2012a, b) also discusses the co-primary endpoint approach for assessing IBS signs and symptoms, using global assessment of symptoms and assessment of symptoms of abdominal discomfort/pain, but they are slightly different from FDA's recommendation. Offen et al. (2007) provide other examples using multiple co-primary endpoints.

The resulting need for new approaches to the design and analysis of clinical trials with multiple endpoints has been noted (Gong et al. 2000; Sankoh et al. 2003; Chuang-Stein et al. 2007; Offen et al. 2007; Hung and Wang 2009; Dmitrienko et al. 2010). Utilizing multiple endpoints may provide the opportunity for characterizing the intervention's multidimensional effects, but also creates challenges.

Specifically controlling Type I and Type II error rates is non-trivial when the multiple endpoints are potentially correlated. When more than one endpoint is viewed as important in a clinical trial, a decision must be made as to whether it is desirable to design the trial to evaluate the joint effects on *all* endpoints or *at least one* of the endpoints. This decision defines the alternative hypothesis to be tested and provides a framework for approaching trial design. When designing the trial to evaluate the joint effects on *all* of the endpoints, no adjustment is needed to control the Type I error rate. The hypothesis associated with each endpoint can be evaluated at the same significance level that is desired for demonstrating effects on all of the endpoints [the International Conference on Harmonisation of Technical Requirements for Registration of Pharmaceuticals for Human Use (ICH) E9 Guideline, 1998; Committee for Proprietary Medical Products, CPMP (2002)]. However, the Type II error rate increases as the number of endpoints to be evaluated increases. This is referred to as "multiple co-primary endpoints" and is related to the intersection–union problem (Offen et al. 2007; Hung and Wang 2009). In contrast, when designing the trial to evaluate an effect on *at least one* of the endpoints, an adjustment is needed to control the Type I error rate. This is referred to as "multiple primary endpoints" or "alternative primary endpoints" and is related to the union–intersection problem (Offen et al. 2007; Hung and Wang 2009; Dmitrienko et al. 2010). The challenges created by multiple co-primary endpoints are several. We discuss some of them here.

Sizing a clinical trial: There is an increasing trend toward requiring that confirmatory clinical trials achieve statistical significance on all of K primary endpoints ($K \geq 2$). Clearly as the number of endpoints increases, it becomes more difficult to achieve statistical significance on all endpoints. This goal requires a sample size adjustment often resulting in a sample size that is too large and impractical to conduct the clinical trial.

One alternative to multiple endpoints is to define a single composite endpoint based on the multiple endpoints. This effectively reduces the problem to a single dimension, thus simplifying the design by avoiding the multiplicity issues associated with multiple endpoints. However, the creation and interpretation of a composite endpoint can be challenging, particularly when treatment effects vary across components with very different levels of clinical importance (Cordoba et al. 2010).

Another method for providing a more practical sample size is to consider incorporating the correlations among the endpoints into the sample size calculation. This has been discussed in fixed-sample designs by many authors (Xiong et al. 2005; Chuang-Stein et al. 2007; Offen et al. 2007; Senn and Bretz 2007; Hung and Wang 2009; Li 2009; Song 2009; Kordzakhia et al. 2010; Sozu et al. 2010, 2011, 2012, 2015; Julious and McIntyre 2012; Sugimoto et al. 2012, 2013; Hamasaki et al. 2013). The correlations among the endpoints may be estimated using data from external or pilot studies although such data are often limited. Inaccurate assumptions regarding the correlations during sample size calculation may affect decision-making in clinical trials. For example, if the correlation is overestimated, then the calculated sample size is too small to detect the joint effect on all the endpoints with the desired power.

Relaxing a rejection region: The corresponding rejection region of the null hypothesis defined as the intersection of K regions associated with the K co-primary endpoints is considerably restricted, resulting in the conservative hypothesis testing, especially when the number of endpoints to be evaluated is large. There is a need for methods' development for relaxing the rejection region. Chuang-Stein et al. (2007) and Kordzakhia et al. (2010) discussed methods to control the Type I error rate. Their strategy is to adjust the significance levels depending on the correlation among the endpoints. The methods may reduce the required sample sizes but introduces other complexities. For example, the sample size calculated to detect the joint effect may be smaller than the sample size calculated for each individual endpoint. The correlation is usually unknown, and assumptions regarding the correlation may be incorrect. This calls into question of how such assumptions regarding the correlation may affect the decision-making in clinical trials.

1.1.2   Non-inferiority

The most fundamental design is the *placebo-controlled trial* in which eligible study participants are randomized to the intervention or a placebo/sham (an inert "fake" intervention). Study participants are then followed over time, and results from the two randomized arms are compared. If the intervention arm can be shown to be more effective or *superior* than the placebo arm, then the effect of the intervention has been demonstrated. Although the placebo-controlled trial is considered the optimal design to scientifically evaluate the benefit–risk profile of an intervention, the use of placebo may be unethical due to the availability of an intervention that has been shown to have a favorable benefit–risk profile (Rothmann et al. 2011).

Non-inferiority (NI) trial designs (sometimes inaccurately referred to as "equivalence trials") have been developed to address this issue. In recent years, NI trials have received a great deal of attention by regulatory authorities (CHMP 2006; FDA 2010a) as well as in the clinical trials' literature. The rationale for NI trials is that in order to appropriately evaluate an intervention, a comparison with a control group is necessary to put the results of an intervention arm into context. However, for some medical indications, randomization to a placebo is unethical due to the availability of a proven effective intervention. In this case, an existing effective intervention may be selected to be an *active* control group (referred to as *active-controlled trials* in contrast to placebo-controlled trials) with the objective to evaluate NI of the test intervention relative to the active control (in contrast to superiority to a placebo control).

The objective of a NI trial is different than a placebo-controlled trial. No longer is it necessary to evaluate whether the test intervention is *superior* (deemed *superiority trials*) to the control as in placebo-controlled trials. Instead, it may be desirable to evaluate whether the test intervention is "at least as good as" or "no worse than" (i.e., non-inferior to) the active control. Thus, it is important to remember that in this context "non-inferiority" does not simply mean "not inferior," but rather "not too inferior" (i.e., differences are smaller than a prespecified margin (Blackwelder 2002). Ideally, the test intervention is better than the active control in other ways (e.g., less expensive, better safety profile, better quality of life, or more convenient or less invasive to administer such as requiring fewer pills or a shorter treatment duration resulting in better adherence). For example, in the treatment of HIV, researchers seek less complicated or less toxic antiretroviral regimens that can display similar efficacy to existing regimens.

NI trials have several complexities, thus requiring careful design, monitoring, analyses, and reporting and publication of results (Snappin 2000; Power et al. 2005; Fleming 2008; Power 2008; Evans 2009; Hamasaki and Evans 2013; Evans and Follmann 2015). We discuss some of the challenges here.

Constancy and assay sensitivity: Two important assumptions associated with the design of NI trials are constancy and assay sensitivity (AS) (ICH 2000; D'Agostino et al. 2003; FDA 2010a). In NI trials, an active control is selected because it has been shown to be efficacious (e.g., superior to placebo) in a completed trial. The constancy assumption states that the observed effect of the active control over placebo in the completed trial would be the same as the effect in the current trial presuming a placebo group was included. This may not be the case if there were differences in trial conduct (e.g., differences in treatment administration, endpoints, or population) between the historical and current trials or if resistance to the control intervention has developed over time (e.g., antibiotic resistance). This assumption is not testable in a trial without a concurrent placebo group.

AS is another important assumption in the design of NI trials. The assumption of AS states that the trial is designed in such a way that it is able to detect differences between therapies if they indeed exist. Unless the instrument that is measuring intervention response is sensitive enough to detect differences, the therapies will display similar responses due to the insensitivity of the instrument, possibly resulting in an inability to detect important differences and to erroneously conclude NI. The endpoints that are selected, how they are measured, and the conduct and integrity of the trial can affect AS.

Selecting a control intervention: A control intervention in a NI trial should be considered carefully. Regulatory approval does not necessarily imply that a therapy can be used as a control. The active control ideally will have clinical efficacy that is (1) of substantial magnitude, (2) estimated with precision in the relevant setting in which the NI trial is being conducted, and (3) preferably quantified in multiple trials. Since the effect size of the active control relative to placebo is used to guide the selection of the NI margin (described later), superiority to placebo must be reliably established and measured. A comprehensive synthesis of the evidence that supports the effect size of the active control (i.e., superiority to placebo) and the NI margin should be assembled. For these reasons, the data may not support a NI design for some indications. When selecting the active control for a NI trial, one must consider how the efficacy of the active control was established (e.g., by showing NI to another active control vs. by showing superiority to placebo). If the active control was shown to be effective via a NI trial, then one must consider the concern for biocreep. Biocreep is the tendency for a slightly inferior therapy (but within the margin of NI) that was shown to be efficacious via a NI trial, to be the active control in the next generation of NI trials (D'Agostino et al. 2003). Multiple generations of NI trials using active controls that were themselves shown to be effective via NI trials could eventually result in the demonstration of the NI of a therapy that is not better than placebo. NI is not transitive: If A is non-inferior to B and B is non-inferior to C, then it does not necessarily follow that A is non-inferior to C. For this reason, some believe that NI trials should generally include the best available active controls.

Selecting a NI margin: The selection of the NI margin in NI trials is a complex issue and one that has created much discussion. In general, the selection of the NI margin is conducted in the design stage of the trial and is utilized to help determine the sample size. Defining the NI margin in NI trials is context-dependent, and it plays a direct role in the interpretation of the trial results.

The selection of the NI margin is partly subjective but also guided by prior data, requiring a combination of statistical reasoning and clinical judgment. Conceptually, one may view the NI margin as the "maximum treatment difference that is clinically irrelevant" or the "largest efficacy difference that is acceptable to sacrifice in order to gain the advantages of the intervention." Selection of the NI often requires interactions between statisticians and clinicians. Since one indirect goal of a NI trial is to show that intervention is superior to placebo, some of the effect of active control over placebo needs to be retained (often termed "preserving a fraction of the effect"). Thus, the NI margin should be selected to be smaller than the effect size of the active control over placebo. Researchers should review the historical data that demonstrated the superiority of the active control to placebo to aid in defining the NI margin. Researchers must also consider the within- and across-trial variability in these estimates (i.e., the uncertainty associated with these estimates). Ideally, the NI margin should be chosen independent of study power, but practical limitations may arise since the selection of NI margin can dramatically affect study power.

A natural question is whether a NI margin can be changed after trial initiation. In general, there is little concern regarding a decrease in the NI margin. However, increasing the NI margin can be perceived as manipulation unless appropriately justified (i.e., based on external data that are independent of the trial).

Analyzing a NI trial: In superiority studies, an ITT-based analysis tends to be conservative (i.e., there is a tendency to underestimate true treatment differences). As a result, ITT-based analysis is generally considered the primary analyses in superiority trials as this helps to protect the Type I error rate. Since the goal of NI trials is to show NI or similarity, an underestimate of the true treatment difference can bias toward NI, thus inflating the "false-positive" Type I error rate (i.e., incorrectly claiming NI). Thus, ITT-based analysis is not necessarily conservative in NI trials. For these reasons, an ITT-based analyses and a per protocol set (PPS)-based analyses (i.e., an analysis based on study participants that adhered to protocol) are often considered as co-primary analyses in NI trials (ICH 1998; D'Agostino et al. 2003). It is important to conduct both analyses (and perhaps additional sensitivity analyses) to assess the robustness of the trial result (CPMP 2000; Evans 2009; Evans and Follmann 2015). PPS-based analyses often result in a larger effect size since ITT-based analysis often dilutes the estimate of the effect, but frequently result in wider confidence intervals since it is based on fewer study participants than ITT-based analysis.

1.1.3 Adaptive Designs

Current medical product development for pharmaceuticals and medical devices suffers from high clinical trial costs and a high risk of the failure. Clinical trial designs with adaptive features (adaptive designs) have the potential to streamline clinical trials making them more efficient, i.e., offering potentially fewer required trial to participants, shortening the duration of clinical trials, and reducing costs. Referring to the FDA guidance on "*Adaptive Design Clinical Trials for Drugs and Biologics*" (FDA 2010b) and "*Adaptive Designs for Medical Device Clinical Studies*" (FDA 2015), a clinical trial design with adaptive features is defined as a study including a prospectively planned opportunity for modification of one or more specified aspects of the study design and hypotheses based on the analysis of accumulated data during the study, where the analyses of the accumulating study data are performed at prospectively planned interims within the study. Analyses can be performed in a fully blinded manner or in an unblinded manner and can occur with or without formal statistical hypothesis testing.

During the last several decades, there has been great interest in conducting clinical trials with adaptive features, especially in medical product development (Gallo et al. 2006). Considerable research and applications of such clinical trial designs have been performed by the pharmaceutical industry and regulatory authorities (Bauer et al. 2016). CHMP (2007), and FDA (2010b, 2015) issued the guidance on an appropriate use of clinical trial designs for drug and biologics that can allow for preplanned trial adaptations implemented based on accumulated data while maintaining the trial validity. The concept of clinical trials with adaptive features could trace back to the 1960s–1970s when adaptive randomization and a class of designs for sequential clinical trials were introduced (Armitage et al. 1969; Zelen 1969; Pocock 1977; Wei 1978; Wei and Durham 1978; O'Brien and Fleming 1979; Slud and Wei 1982; Lan and DeMets 1983). In these conventional and classical group-sequential clinical trials, accumulating data are monitored periodically in a trial and the trial is terminated as soon as there has been sufficient evidence to reach a conclusion on either of a positive result (early stopping for efficacy) or of a negative outcome (early stopping for futility).

In recent clinical trials, there has been considerable interest in the use of modern adaptive designs. Modern adaptive designs are often defined by characteristics such as sample size recalculation, enrichment and subgroup identification, and treatment or dose selection (Bauer and Köhne 1994; Proschan and Hunsberger 1995; Fisher 1998; Cui et al. 1999; Lehmacher and Wassmer 1999; Müller and Schäfer 2001; Tsiatis and Mehta 2003; Chen et al. 2004; Mehta et al. 2007). The use of modern adaptive design in clinical trials can create opportunities for saving resources, reducing risk of project failure, and improving productivity. For more details on the recent developments in clinical trial designs with adaptive features in clinical trials, see Bauer et al. (2016).

Clinical trial designs with adaptive features can allow for modifying the characteristics of a trial based on cumulative information at an interim point of the trial. FDA guidance on adaptive designs for drug and biologics (FDA 2010b, 2015) indicates that the possible changes or modification in design or analyses are as follows:

- Eligibility criteria (either for subsequent study enrollment or for a subset selection of an analytic population);
- Randomization procedure (methods and allocation ratio);
- Treatment regimens of the study groups (e.g., dose level, schedule, or duration);
- Sample size (including early termination);
- Concomitant treatment use;
- Schedule of evaluations (e.g., number of intermediate time points, timing of last patient observation, and duration of study participation);
- Primary endpoints (e.g., type of outcome assessments, time point of assessment, use of a unitary versus composite endpoint or the components included in a composite endpoint);
- Selection and/or order of secondary endpoints;
- Analysis methods (e.g., covariates of final analysis, statistical methodology, Type I error control).

These changes or modifications must be fully described and documented in both of the protocol and of the statistical analysis plan.

Adaptive designs have the following advantages:

- Uncertainty can be reduced. This may lead to an improvement in trial design by getting additional information from the ongoing trial.
- Better information is obtained on the intervention, resulting in a reduced probability that the phase III dose will either be toxic or show inadequate efficacy.
- Ethical benefits to patients through early dropping of doses that are ineffective or harmful and earlier switching to doses that provide therapeutic benefit.

However, there are also issues that must be considered carefully including the following:

- Appropriate rationale for adaptive designs: Why and how.
- Control of Type I error: Bias that increases the chance of a false conclusion that a test intervention is effective.
- Adaptations well defined in advance.

- Protocol for interim monitoring known in advance.
- Appropriate firewalls in place to maintain appropriate blinding of accumulating study results.
- After-the-fact proof that the protocol and interim monitoring procedures were followed (audit capability).

1.2 Organization of the Book

Many recent clinical trials for evaluating efficacy and safety of new interventions include multiple objectives, especially in medical product development. There are advantages of clinical trials with multiple objectives over trials with a single objective saving time and resources and more completely characterizing the intervention effects. However, such clinical trials require conducting a number of statistical tests and analyses associated with multiple objectives, and then, complex multiplicity or multiple testing problems occur (Huque et al. 2013). During the last several years, our team has conducted research on the design and analysis of such clinical trials, especially focusing on group-sequential designs for clinical trials with multiple objectives. Since the early application of group-sequential designs into clinical trials, e.g., BHAT [Beta Blocker Heart Attack Trial Research Group (1982), which is the first large-scale multicenter trial to use the O'Brien and Fleming method (Halperin et al. 1990)], there have been many successful stories in the use of group-sequential designs in clinical trials (DeMets et al. 2006; Hung et al. 2015). We have especially focused on clinical trial designs with co-objectives including multiple co-primary endpoints and three-arm NI designs evaluating assay sensitivity and NI, in a confirmatory clinical trial setting (Asakura et al. 2014, 2015a, b; Ando et al. 2015; Hamasaki et al. 2015; Ochiai et al. 2016).

This book summarizes the results of our research in an integrated manner for the purpose of helping statisticians involved in clinical trials understand these methodologies. The book focuses on group-sequential designs in (i) superiority clinical trials for comparing the effect of two interventions with multiple endpoints and (ii) three-arm NI clinical trials for evaluating AS from the perspective of evaluation of the control intervention relative to placebo and NI of the test intervention to control intervention. For clinical trials with multiple endpoints, we focus on a situation where the alternative hypothesis is that there are effects on *all* endpoints in a group-sequential setting. We only briefly discuss trials designed with an alternative hypothesis of an effect on *at least one* endpoint with a prespecified non-ordering of endpoints.

The structure of the book is as follows: In Chap. 2, we describe the group-sequential designs for early efficacy stopping in superiority clinical trials comparing the effect of two interventions with two co-primary endpoints. We discuss two situations based on the endpoint scales, i.e., (i) both endpoints are continuous and (ii) both endpoints are binary. We derive the power and sample size within two decision-making frameworks. One framework is to conclude the test intervention's benefit relative to control when superiority is achieved for the two endpoints at the same interim time point of the trial. The other framework is when superiority is achieved for the two endpoints at any interim time point, not necessarily simultaneously. We evaluate the behavior of the required sample size, power, and Type I error as design parameters (standardized mean differences, the number of planned analyses, and efficacy critical boundaries) vary. We provide an example to illustrate the methods and discuss practical considerations when designing efficient group-sequential designs in clinical trials with co-primary endpoints.

In Chap. 3, we discuss sample size recalculation based on the observed intervention's effects at an interim analysis with a focus on control of the statistical error rates. Clinical trials are designed based on assumptions often constructed based on prior data. However, prior data may be limited or an inaccurate indication of future data, resulting in trials that are over/underpowered. Interim analyses provide an opportunity to evaluate the accuracy of the design assumptions and potentially make design adjustments if the assumptions were markedly inaccurate. We consider the sample size recalculation based on the two decision-making frameworks discussed in Chap. 2.

In Chap. 4, as an extension of the methods discussed in Chap. 2, we describe the group-sequential designs for early efficacy or futility stopping in superiority clinical trials comparing the effect of two interventions with two co-primary endpoints. We describe several decision-making frameworks for evaluating efficacy or futility, based on boundaries using group-sequential methodology. We incorporate the correlations among the endpoints into the calculations for futility critical boundaries and sample sizes. We provide an example to illustrate the methods.

In Chap. 5, we provide an overview of the concepts and technical fundamentals regarding group-sequential designs for clinical trials with two primary endpoints. There are many procedures for controlling the Type I error rate. We discuss a common and simple procedure, i.e., the weighted Bonferroni procedure. We evaluate the behavior of the sample size, power, and Type I error rate associated with the procedure.

In Chap. 6, we discuss group-sequential three-arm NI clinical trial designs that include active and placebo controls for evaluating both AS and NI. We extend two existing approaches, the fixed margin and fraction approaches, into a group-sequential setting with two decision-making frameworks. We provide an example to illustrate the methods.

This aggregation of the work provides a foundation for designing randomized trials with other design features including clinical trials with more than two interventions (dose selection clinical trials), trials with time-to-event endpoints, trials with targeted subgroups, and multiregional clinical trials. In Chap. 7, we describe briefly issues in designing such trials.

The book assumes that the readers have enough knowledge on group-sequential designs with a single objective. For the fundamentals, see Whitehead (1997), Jennison and Turnbull (2000), DeMets et al. (2006), and Proschan et al. (2006).

References

Ando Y, Hamasaki T, Evans SR, Asakura K, Sugimoto T, Sozu T, Ohno Y (2015) Sample size considerations in clinical trials when comparing two interventions using multiple co-primary binary relative risk contrasts. Stat Biopharm Res 7:81–94

Armitage P, McPherson CK, Rowe BC (1969) Repeated significance test on accumulating data. J Roy Stat Soc A132:235–244

Asakura K, Hamasaki T, Sugimoto T, Hayashi K, Evans SR, Sozu T (2014) Sample size determination in group-sequential clinical trials with two co-primary endpoints. Stat Med 33:2897–2913

Asakura K, Hamasaki T, Evans SR (2015a) Interim evaluation of efficacy or futility in group-sequential clinical trials with multiple co-primary endpoints. The 2015 Joint Statistical Meetings, Seattle, USA, 8–13 August

Asakura K, Hamasaki T, Evans SR, Sugimoto T, Sozu T (2015b) Sample size determination in group-sequential clinical trials with two co-primary endpoints. In: Chen Z, Liu A, Qu Y, Tang L, Ting N, Tsong Y (eds) Applied statistics in bio-medicine and clinical trial design (Chapter 14). Springer International Publishing, Cham/Heidelberg/New York, pp 235–262

Bauer P, Köhne K (1994) Evaluation of experiments with adaptive interim analyses. Biometrics 50:1029–1041 (correction in Biometrics 1996, 52:380)

Bauer P, Bretz F, Dragalin V, König F, Wassmer G (2016) Twenty-five years of confirmatory adaptive designs: opportunities and pitfalls. Stat Med 35:325–347

Beta-Blocker Heart Attack Trial Research Group (1982) A randomized trial of propranolol in patients with acute myocardial infraction: I. Motility results. J Am Med Assoc 247:1707–1714

Blackwelder WC (2002) Showing a treatment is good because it is not bad: when does "noninferiority" imply effectiveness. Control Clin Trials 23:52–54

Chen YHJ, DeMets DL, Lan KKG (2004) Increasing the sample size when the unblinded interim results is promising. Stat Med 23:1023–1038

Chuang-Stein C, Stryszak P, Dmitrienko A, Offen W (2007) Challenge of multiple co-primary endpoints: a new approach. Stat Med 26:1181–1192

Committee for Medicinal Products for Human Use (2007) Reflection paper on methodological issues in confirmatory clinical trials planned with an adaptive design (CHMP/EWP/2459/02). European Medicines Agency, London, UK. Available at: http://www.ema.europa.eu/docs/en_GB/document_library/Scientific_guideline/2009/09/WC500003616.pdf. Accessed 25 Nov 2015

Committee for Medicinal Products for Human Use (2008) Guideline on medicinal products for the treatment Alzheimer's disease and other dementias (CPMP/EWP/553/95 Rev.1). European Medicines Agency, London, UK. Available at: http://www.ema.europa.eu/docs/en_GB/document_library/Scientific_guideline/2009/09/WC500003562.pdf. Accessed 25 Nov 2015

Committee for Medicinal Products for Human Use (2012a) Guideline on clinical investigation of medicinal products for the treatment of acute heart failure (CHMP/EWP/2986/03 Rev.1). European Medical Agency, London, UK. Available at: http://www.ema.europa.eu/docs/en_GB/document_library/Scientific_guideline/2015/06/WC500187797.pdf. Accessed 25 Nov 2015

Committee for Medicinal Products for Human Use (2012b) Guideline on clinical investigation of medicinal products in the treatment or prevention of diabetes mellitus (CPMP/EWP/1080/00 Rev.1). European Medical Agency, London, UK. Available at: http://www.ema.europa.eu/docs/en_GB/document_library/Scientific_guideline/2012/06/WC500129256.pdf. Accessed 25 Nov 2015

Committee for Medicinal Products for Human Use (2013a) Draft guideline on the clinical investigation of medicinal products for the treatment of duchenne and becker muscular dystrophy (EMA/CHMP/236981/2011). European Medical Agency, London, UK. Available at: http://www.ema.europa.eu/docs/en_GB/document_library/Scientific_guideline/2013/03/WC500139508.pdf. Accessed 25 Nov 2015

Committee for Medicinal Products for Human Use (2013b) Guideline on the evaluation of medicinal products for the treatment of irritable bowel syndrome (CPMP/EWP/785/97 Rev.1, 27). European Medical Agency, London, UK. Available at: http://www.ema.europa.eu/docs/en_GB/document_library/Scientific_guideline/2014/09/WC500173457.pdf. Accessed 25 Nov 2015

Committee for Medicinal Products for Human Use European Medicines Agency (2006) Guideline on the choice of the non-inferiority margin. Stat Med 25:1628–1638

Committee for Proprietary Medical Products (2000) Points to consider on switching between superiority and non-inferiority. CPMP/EWP/482/99. European Medicines Agency, London, UK. Available at: http://www.ema.europa.eu/docs/en_GB/document_library/Scientific_guideline/2009/09/WC500003658.pdf. Accessed 25 Nov 2015

Committee for Proprietary Medical Products (2002) Points to consider on multiplicity issues in clinical trials (CPMP/EWP/908/99). European Medicines Agency, London, UK. Available at: http://www.ema.europa.eu/docs/en_GB/document_library/Scientific_guideline/2009/09/WC500003640.pdf. Accessed 25 Nov 2015

Cordoba G, Schwartz L, Woloshin S, Bae H, Gøtzsche PC (2010) Definition, reporting, and interpretation of composite outcomes in clinical trials: systematic review. Br Med J 341:c3920

Cui L, Hung HMJ, Wang SJ (1999) Modification of sample size in group sequential clinical trials. Biometrics 55:853–857

D'Agostino RB, Massaro JM, Sullivan LM (2003) Non-inferiority trials: design concepts and issues—the encounters of academic consultants in statistics. Stat Med 22:169–186

DeMets D, Furberg CD, Friedman LM (2006) Data monitoring in clinical trials: a case studies approach. Springer, New York

Dmitrienko A, Tamhane AC, Bretz F (2010) Multiple testing problems in pharmaceutical statistics. Chapman and Hall/CRC, Boca Raton

Evans SR (2009) Noninferiority clinical trials. Chance 22:53–58

Evans SR, Follmann D (2015) Fundamentals and innovation in antibiotic trials. Stat Biopharm Res 7:331–336

Evans SR, Ting N (2015) Fundamental concepts for new clinical trialists. Chapman and Hall/CRC Press, Boca Raton

Fisher LD (1998) Self-designing clinical trials. Stat Med 17:1551–1562

Fleming TR (2008) Current issues in non-inferiority trials. Stat Med 27:317–332

Food and Drug Administration (2006) Critical path opportunities list. U.S. Department of Health and Human Services Food and Drug Administration, Rockville, MD, USA

Food and Drug Administration (2010a) Guidance for industry: non-inferiority clinical trials (draft guidance). U.S. Department of Health and Human Services Food and Drug Administration, Rockville, MD, USA. Available at: http://www.fda.gov/ucm/groups/fdagov-public/@fdagov-drugs-gen/documents/document/ucm202140.pdf. Accessed 25 Nov 2015

Food and Drug Administration (2010b) Guidance for industry: adaptive design clinical trials for drugs and biologics. U.S. Department of Health and Human Services Food and Drug Administration, Rockville, MD, USA. Available at: http://www.fda.gov/downloads/Drugs/Guidances/ucm201790.pdf. Accessed 25 Nov 2015

Food and Drug Administration (2012) Guidance for industry: irritable bowel syndrome: clinical evaluation of products for treatment. U.S. Department of Health and Human Services Food and Drug Administration, Rockville, MD, USA. Available at: http://www.fda.gov/ucm/groups/fdagov-public/documents/document/ucm205269.pdf. Accessed 25 Nov 2015

Food and Drug Administration (2013) Guidance for industry: Alzheimer's disease: developing drugs for the treatment of early stage disease. U.S. Department of Health and Human Services Food and Drug Administration, Rockville, MD, USA. Available at: http://www.fda.gov/ucm/groups/fdagov-public/@fdagov-drugs-gen/documents/document/ucm338287.pdf. Accessed 25 Nov 2015

Food and Drug Administration (2015) Draft guidance for industry and food and drug administration staff: adaptive designs for medical device clinical studies. U.S. Department of Health and Human Services Food and Drug Administration, Rockville, MD, USA. Available at: http://www.fda.

gov/ucm/groups/fdagov-public/@fdagov-meddev-gen/documents/document/ucm446729.pdf . Accessed 25 Nov 2015

Gallo P, Chuang-Stein C, Dragalin V, Gaydos B, Krams M, Pinheiro J (2006) PhRMA working group adaptive designs in clinical drug development: an executive summary of the PhRMA working group. J Biopharm Stat 16:275–283

Gong J, Pinheiro JC, DeMets DL (2000) Estimating significance level and power comparisons for testing multiple endpoints in clinical trials. Contr Clin Trials 21:313–329

Halperin M, DeMets DL, Ware JH (1990) Early methodological developments for clinical trials at the National Heart, Lung and Blood Institute. Stat Med 9:881–892

Hamasaki T, Evans SR (2013) Noninferiority clinical trials: issues in design, monitoring, analyses, and reporting. Igaku no Ayumi (J Clin Exp Med) 244:1212–1216 (in Japanese)

Hamasaki T, Sugimoto T, Evans SR, Sozu T (2013) Sample size determination for clinical trials with co-primary outcomes: exponential event times. Pharm Stat 12:28–34

Hamasaki T, Asakura K, Evans SR, Sugimoto T, Sozu T (2015) Group-sequential strategies in clinical trials with multiple co-primary endpoints. Stat Biopharm Res 7:36–54

Hung HMJ, Wang SJ (2009) Some controversial multiple testing problems in regulatory applications. J Biopharm Stat 19:1–11

Hung HMJ, Wang SJ, Yang P, Jin K, Lawrence J, Kordzakhia G, Massie T (2015) Statistical challenges in regulatory review of cardiovascular and CNS clinical trials. J Biopharm Stat (First published online on 14 Sept 2015 as doi:10.1080/10543406.2015.1092025)

Huque MF, Dmitrienko A, D'Agostino R (2013) Multiplicity issues in clinical trials with multiple objectives. Stat Biopharm Res 5:321–337

International Conference on Harmonisation of Technical Requirements for Registration of Pharmaceuticals for Human Use (ICH) (1998) ICH harmonised tripartite guideline E9: statistical principles for clinical trials. February 1998. Available at: http://www.ich.org/fileadmin/Public_Web_Site/ICH_Products/Guidelines/Efficacy/E9/Step4/E9_Guideline.pdf. Accessed 25 Nov 2015

International Conference on Harmonisation of Technical Requirements for Registration of Pharmaceuticals for Human Use (ICH) (2000) ICH harmonised tripartite guideline E10: choice of control group and related issues in clinical trials. July 2000. Available at: http://www.ich.org/fileadmin/Public_Web_Site/ICH_Products/Guidelines/Efficacy/E10/Step4/E10_Guideline.pdf. Accessed 25 Nov 2015

Jennison C, Turnbull BW (2000) Group sequential methods with applications to clinical trials. Chapman and Hall/CRC Press, Boca Raton

Julious S, McIntyre NE (2012) Sample sizes for trials involving multiple correlated must-win comparisons. Pharm Stat 11:177–185

Kordzakhia G, Siddiqui O, Huque MF (2010) Method of balanced adjustment in testing co-primary endpoints. Stat Med 29:2055–2066

Lan KKG, DeMets DL (1983) Discrete sequential boundaries for clinical trials. Biometrika 70:659–663

Lehmacher W, Wassmer G (1999) Adaptive sample size calculations in group sequential trials. Biometrics 55:1286–1290

i QH (2009) Evaluating co-primary endpoints collectively in clinical trials. Biometrical J 51:137–145

Mehta CR, Bauer P, Posch M, Brannath W (2007) Repeated confidence intervals for adaptive group sequential trials. Stat Med 26:5422–5433

Mosteller F (1981) Innovation and evaluation. Science 211:881–886

Müller HH, Schäfer H (2001) Adaptive group sequential designs for clinical trials: combining the advantages of adaptive and of classical group sequential approaches. Biometrics 57:886–891

O'Brien PC, Fleming TR (1979) A multiple testing procedure for clinical trials. Biometrics 35:549–556

Ochiai T, Hamasaki T, Evans SR, Asakura K, Ohno Y (2016) Group-sequential three-arm noninferiority clinical trial designs. J Biopharm Stat (First published online: 18 Feb 2016 as doi:10.1080/10543406.2016.1148710)

Offen W, Chuang-Stein C, Dmitrienko A, Littman G, Maca J, Meyerson L, Muirhead R,
    Stryszak P, Boddy A, Chen K, Copley-Merriman K, Dere W, Givens S, Hall D, Henry D,
    Jackson JD, Krishen A, Liu T, Ryder S, Sankoh AJ, Wang J, Yeh CH (2007) Multiple
    co-primary endpoints: medical and statistical solutions. Drug Inf J 41:31–46
Pocock SJ (1977) Group sequential methods in the design and analysis of clinical trials.
    Biometrika 64:191–199
Powers JH (2008) Noninferiority and equivalence trials: deciphering 'similarity' of medical
    interventions. Stat Med 27:343–352
Powers JH, Cooper CK, Lin D, Ross DB (2005) Sample size and the ethics of non-inferiority
    trials. Lancet 366:24–25
Proschan MA, Hunsberger SA (1995) Designed extension of studies based on conditional power.
    Biometrics 51:1315–1324
Proschan MA, Lan KKG, Wittes JT (2006) Statistical monitoring of clinical trials: a unified
    approach. Springer, New York
Rothmann MD, Wiens BL, Chan ISF (2011) Design and analysis of non-inferiority trials.
    Chapman and Hall/CRC, Boca Raton, FL
Sankoh AJ, D'Agostino RB, Huque MF (2003) Efficacy endpoint selection and multiplicity
    adjustment methods in clinical trials with inherent multiple endpoint issues. Stat Med 22:3133–
    3150
Senn S, Bretz F (2007) Power and sample size when multiple endpoints are considered. Pharm Stat
    6:161–170
Slud EV, Wei LJ (1982) Two-sample repeated significance tests based on the modified Wilcoxon
    statistics. J Am Stat Assoc 77:862–868
Snappin SM (2000) Noninferiority trials. Curr Control Trials Cardiovasc Med 1:19–21
Song JX (2009) Sample size for simultaneous testing of rate differences in noninferiority trials
    with multiple endpoints. Comput Stat Data Anal 53:1201–1207
Sozu T, Sugimoto T, Hamasaki T (2010) Sample size determination in clinical trials with multiple
    co-primary binary endpoints. Stat Med 29:2169–2179
Sozu T, Sugimoto T, Hamasaki T (2011) Sample size determination in superiority clinical trials
    with multiple co-primary correlated endpoints. J Biopharm Stat 21:1–19
Sozu T, Sugimoto T, Hamasaki T (2012) Sample size determination in clinical trials with multiple
    co-primary endpoints including mixed continuous and binary variables. Biometrical J 54:
    716–729
Sozu T, Sugimoto T, Hamasaki T, Evans SR (2015) Sample size determination in clinical trials
    with multiple primary endpoints. Springer International Press, Cham/Heidelberg/New York
Sugimoto T, Sozu T, Hamasaki T (2012) A convenient formula for sample size calculations in
    clinical trials with multiple co-primary continuous endpoints. Pharm Stat 11:118–128
Sugimoto T, Sozu T, Hamasaki T, Evans SR (2013) A logrank test-based method for sizing
    clinical trials with two co-primary time-to-event endpoints. Biostatistics 14:409–421
Tsiatis AA, Mehta C (2003) On the inefficiency of the adaptive design for monitoring clinical
    trials. Biometrika 90:367–378
Wei LJ (1978) The adaptive biased coin design for sequential experiments. Ann Stat 6:92–100
Wei LJ, Durham S (1978) The randomized play-the-winner rule in medical trials. J Am Stat Assoc
    73:840–843
Whitehead J (1997) The design and analysis of sequential clinical trials, revised, 2nd edn. Wiley,
    Chichester
Xiong C, Yu K, Gao F, Yan Y, Zhang Z (2005) Power and sample size for clinical trials when
    efficacy is required in multiple endpoints: application to an Alzheimer's treatment trial. Clin
    Trials 2:387–393
Zelen M (1969) Play the winner rule and the controlled clinical trial. J Am Stat Assoc 64:131–146

Chapter 2
Interim Evaluation of Efficacy in Clinical Trials with Two Co-primary Endpoints

Abstract We discuss group-sequential designs for early efficacy stopping in clinical trials with two outcomes as co-primary endpoints, i.e., trials designed to evaluate whether the test intervention is superior to the control on *all* primary endpoints. We discuss two outcome scale situations: (i) when both outcomes are continuous, and (ii) when both outcomes are binary. We derive the power and sample size formulae within two decision-making frameworks: (A) evaluation of superiority not necessarily simultaneously and (B) evaluation of superiority for the two primary endpoints simultaneously. We evaluate the behaviors of sample size and power with varying design characteristics and provide an example to illustrate the methods.

Keywords Average sample number · Binary outcomes · Continuous outcomes · Efficacy stopping · Lan–DeMets error-spending method · Maximum sample size · O'Brien–Fleming-type boundary · Pocock-type boundary · Type I error · Type II error · Intersection–union test

2.1 Introduction

In this chapter, we describe the methods for designing group-sequential clinical trials with two outcomes as co-primary endpoints, where a trial is designed to evaluate whether the test intervention is superior to the control on *all* primary endpoints, and to be terminated early when evidence is overwhelming (early stopping for efficacy). Group-sequential designs for multiple co-primary endpoints are a more attractive design feature rather than the fixed-sample designs because they offer the possibility of stopping a trial when evidence is overwhelming, thus providing efficiency (Hung and Wang 2009) as the sample size in fixed-sample clinical trials with multiple co-primary endpoints is often unnecessarily large and impractical.

Recently, Asakura et al. (2014, 2015) discussed two decision-making frameworks associated with interim evaluation of efficacy in clinical trials with two co-primary endpoints in a group-sequential setting. One framework is to reject the null hypothesis if and only if statistical significance is achieved for the two endpoints simultaneously (i.e., at the same interim time-point of the trial). The other is a generalization of this, i.e., to reject the null hypothesis if superiority is demonstrated for the two endpoints at any interim time-point (i.e., not necessarily simultaneously). The former framework is independently discussed by Chang et al. (2014) and evaluated in clinical trials with two co-primary endpoints. Hamasaki et al. (2015) discussed more flexible decision-making frameworks, allowing the different time-points of analyses among the endpoints. In addition, Jennison and Turnbull (1993) and Cook and Farewell (1994) discussed the decision-making frameworks associated with interim evaluation of efficacy and futility to monitor the efficacy and safety responses and considered a simple method for determining the boundaries as if the responses are not correlated (i.e., assuming zero correlations between the responses). The methods for the interim evaluation of efficacy and futility will be discussed in Chap. 4.

We discuss two outcome scale situations: (i) when both outcomes are continuous (in Sect. 2.2) and (ii) when both outcomes are binary (Sect. 2.3). We derive the power and sample size formulae within two decision-making frameworks for early efficacy stopping: (A) evaluation of superiority not necessarily simultaneously and (B) evaluation of superiority for the two primary endpoints simultaneously. We evaluate the behaviors of sample size and power with varying design characteristics and provide an example to illustrate the methods. For more than two endpoints, see Hamasaki et al. (2015).

2.2 Continuous Outcomes

2.2.1 Notation and Statistical Setting

Consider a randomized, group-sequential clinical trial of comparing the test intervention (T) with the control intervention (C). Two continuous outcomes (i.e., $K = 2$), EP1 and EP2, are to be evaluated as co-primary endpoints. Suppose that a maximum of L analyses is planned, where the same number of planned analyses with the same information space is selected for both endpoints. Let n_l and $r_C n_l$ be the cumulative number of participants on the T and the C at the lth analysis ($l = 1, \ldots, L$), respectively, where r_C is the allocation ratio of the C to the T. Hence, up to n_L and $r_C n_L$ participants are recruited and randomly assigned to the T and the C, respectively. Then, there are n_L paired outcomes (Y_{T1i}, Y_{T2i}) $(i = 1, \ldots, n_L)$ for the T and $r_C n_L$ paired outcomes (Y_{C1j}, Y_{C2j}) $(j = 1, \ldots, r_C n_L)$ for the C. Assume that (Y_{T1i}, Y_{T2i}) and (Y_{C1j}, Y_{C2j}) are independently bivariate distributed with means $E[Y_{Tki}] = \mu_{Tk}$ and $E[Y_{Ckj}] = \mu_{Ck}$, variances $var[Y_{Tki}] = \sigma_{Tk}^2$ and $var[Y_{Ckj}] = \sigma_{Ck}^2$, and correlation $corr[Y_{T1i}, Y_{T2i}] = \rho_T$ and $corr[Y_{C1j}, Y_{C2j}] = \rho_C$, respectively ($k = 1, 2$). For simplicity, the variances are assumed to be known and common, i.e., $\sigma_{Tk}^2 = \sigma_{Ck}^2 = \sigma_k^2$. Note that the method can be applied to the case of unknown variances. For the fixed-sample designs, Sozu et al. (2011) discuss a method for the unknown variance case and show that the calculated sample size is nearly equivalent to that for the known variance in the setting of 80 % or 90 % power at 2.5 % significance level for one-sided test. By analogy from the fixed-sample designs, there may be no practical difference in the group-sequential setting and the methodology for a known variance provides a reasonable approximation for the unknown variances case.

Let $\delta_k = \mu_{Tk} - \mu_{Ck}$ and $\Delta_k = \delta_k / \sigma_k$ denote the mean differences and standardized mean differences for the T and the C, respectively ($k = 1, 2$). Suppose that positive values of δ_k represent the test intervention's benefit. There is an interest in conducting a one-sided hypothesis test at the significance level of α to evaluate whether the T is superior to the C on both endpoints. The hypothesis for each endpoint is tested at significance level of α: The hypotheses are H_{0k}: $\delta_k \leq 0$ versus H_{1k}: $\delta_k > 0$. For multiple co-primary endpoints, "success" can be declared if the superiority is achieved on both endpoints. The hypotheses for co-primary endpoints are the null hypothesis H_0: $H_{01} \cup H_{02}$ versus the alternative hypothesis (the union H_0 of both individual nulls is tested against the intersection alternative H_1: $H_{11} \cap H_{12}$). This is referred to as the intersection–union test (Berger 1982).

Let (Z_{1l}, Z_{2l}) be the statistics for testing the hypotheses at the lth analysis, given by

$$Z_{kl} = \frac{\bar{Y}_{Tkl} - \bar{Y}_{Ckl}}{\sigma_k \sqrt{(1 + 1/r_C)/n_l}},$$

where $\bar{Y}_{Tkl}$ and $\bar{Y}_{Ckl}$ are the sample means given by $\bar{Y}_{Tkl} = \sum_{i=1}^{n_l} Y_{Tki}/n_l$ and $\bar{Y}_{Ckl} = \sum_{j=1}^{r_C n_l} Y_{Ckj}/(r_C n_l)$. For large samples, under the alternative hypothesis H_1, each Z_{kl} is approximately normally distributed as $Z_{kl} \sim N(\sqrt{r_C n_l/(1 + r_C)}\delta_k/\sigma_k, 1^2)$. Thus, (Z_{1l}, Z_{2l}) is approximately bivariate normally distributed with the correlation $\text{corr}[Z_{1l}, Z_{2l}] = (r_C \rho_T + \rho_C)/(1 + r_C) = \rho_Z$ at the lth interim analysis. Furthermore, the joint distribution of $(Z_{11}, Z_{21}, \ldots, Z_{1l}, Z_{2l}, \ldots, Z_{1L}, Z_{2L})$ is $2L$ multivariate normal with their correlations given by $\text{corr}[Z_{1l'}, Z_{1l}] = \text{corr}[Z_{2l'}, Z_{2l}] = \sqrt{n_{l'}/n_l}$, and $\text{corr}[Z_{1l'}, Z_{2l}] = \text{corr}[Z_{1l}, Z_{2l'}] = \rho_Z \sqrt{n_{l'}/n_l}$, where $1 \leq l' \leq l \leq L$ and $k' \leq k$. If the correlation between the two endpoints is assumed be common between the two intervention groups, i.e., $\rho_T = \rho_C = \rho$, then the correlation among test statistics across the interim analyses is simply given by $\text{corr}[Z_{1l'}, Z_{2l}] = \text{corr}[Z_{1l}, Z_{2l'}] = \rho \sqrt{n_{l'}/n_l}$ as $\rho_Z = \rho$.

2.2.2 Decision-Making Frameworks and Stopping Rules

When evaluating the joint effects on both of the endpoints within the context of group-sequential designs, there are the two decision-making frameworks associated with hypothesis testing. One is to reject H_0 if statistical significance of T relative to C is achieved for both endpoints at any interim analysis until the final analysis (i.e., not necessarily simultaneously at the same interim analysis) (DF-A) (Asakura et al. 2014), and the other is the special case of DF-A and is to reject H_0 if and only if superiority is achieved for the two endpoints simultaneously (i.e., at the same interim analysis of the trial) (DF-B) (Asakura et al. 2014; Cheng et al. 2014). We will discuss the two decision-making frameworks separately as the corresponding stopping rules and power definitions are unique.

DF-A is flexible. If only the hypothesis for one endpoint is rejected at an interim analysis, then the trial will continue but in subsequent interim analyses the not-yet-rejected hypothesis for other endpoint is repeatedly tested until it is rejected or the trial is completed. The stopping rule based on DF-A is formally given as follows:

At the lth analysis $(l = 1, \ldots, L - 1)$

if $Z_{1l} > c_{1l}^E(\alpha)$ and $Z_{2l'} > c_{2l'}^E(\alpha)$ for some $1 \leq l' \leq l$, or if $Z_{1l'} > c_{1l'}^E(\alpha)$ for some $1 \leq l' \leq l$ and $Z_{2l} > c_{2l}^E(\alpha)$, then reject H_0 and stop the trial, otherwise, continue the $(l+1)$th analysis,

at the Lth analysis

if $Z_{1L} > c_{1L}^E(\alpha)$ and $Z_{2l'} > c_{2l'}^E(\alpha)$ for some $1 \leq l' \leq L$, or if $Z_{1l'} > c_{1l'}^E(\alpha)$ for some $1 \leq l' \leq L$ and $Z_{2L} > c_{2L}^E(\alpha)$, then reject H_0 and stop the trial, otherwise, then do not reject H_0,

where $c_{1l}^E(\alpha)$ and $c_{2l}^E(\alpha)$ are the critical boundaries, which are constant and selected separately, using any group-sequential method such as the Lan–DeMets error-spending method (Lan and DeMets 1983) to control the overall Type I error rate, as if they were a single primary endpoint, ignoring the other co-primary endpoint.

For example, consider a group-sequential clinical trial with the five planned analyses $(L = 5)$. The hypothesis for the joint effect on both endpoints is tested at 2.5 % significance level. If the critical boundaries for both endpoints are commonly determined by the O'Brien–Fleming-type boundary (OF) (O'Brien and Fleming 1979), using the Lan–DeMets error-spending method with equally spaced increments of information, then critical boundaries for each analysis are 4.8769, 3.3569, 2.6803, 2.2898, and 2.0310. Figure 2.1 illustrates the region for rejecting each H_{0k} $(k = 1, 2)$. For example, if we observe the test statistics $Z_{14} = 3.5073$ for EP1 and $Z_{24} = 2.2294$ for EP2 at the fourth analysis, then H_0 is not rejected as Z_{14} is larger than the corresponding critical boundary of $c_{14}^E(2.5) = 2.2898$ but Z_{24} is not. In the subsequent analysis, i.e., the final analysis, the hypothesis testing is repeatedly conducted only for EP2. At the final analysis, if we observe $Z_{25} = 2.9732$ for EP2, then H_0 is rejected as Z_{25} is larger than the corresponding critical boundary of $c_{25}^E(2.5) = 2.0310$.

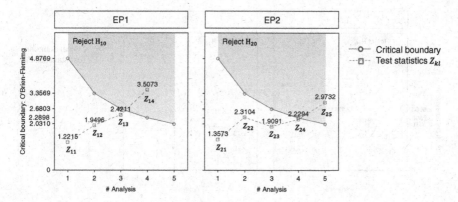

Fig. 2.1 The region for rejecting H_0 based on DF-A in a group-sequential clinical trial with the five planned analyses ($L = 5$), where the decision-making is based on DF-A. The hypothesis for the joint effect on both endpoints is tested at 2.5 % significance level. The critical boundaries for both endpoints are commonly determined by the OF, using the Lan–DeMets error-spending method with equally spaced increments of information

The power for the joint effect on both endpoints, corresponding to DF-A, is

$$1 - \beta = \Pr\left[\left\{\bigcup_{l=1}^{L} A_{1l}\right\} \cap \left\{\bigcup_{l=1}^{L} A_{2l}\right\}\middle| H_1\right], \tag{2.1}$$

where $A_{kl} = \left\{Z_{kl} > c_{kl}^{\mathrm{E}}\right\}$. The power based on DF-A (2.1) can be numerically assessed by using multivariate normal integrals. A detailed calculation is provided in Appendix A.

DF-B is relatively simple. If only the hypothesis for one endpoint is rejected at an interim analysis, then the trial continues and the hypotheses for both endpoints are repeatedly tested until they are rejected simultaneously, i.e., during the same interim analysis. The stopping rule based on DF-B is formally given as follows:

At the lth analysis ($l = 1, \ldots, L - 1$)

if $Z_{1l} > c_{1l}^{\mathrm{E}}(\alpha)$ and $Z_{2l} > c_{2l}^{\mathrm{E}}(\alpha)$, then reject H_0 and stop the trial, otherwise, continue to the $(l + 1)$th analysis,

at the Lth analysis

if $Z_{1L} > c_{1L}^{\mathrm{E}}(\alpha)$ and $Z_{2L} > c_{2L}^{\mathrm{E}}(\alpha)$, then reject H_0, otherwise, do not reject H_0.

Figure 2.2 illustrates the region for rejecting each H_{k0} with the number of planned analyses similarly as in Fig. 2.1. For example, if we observe the test

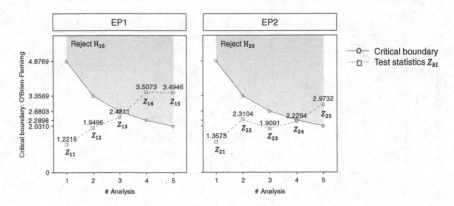

Fig. 2.2 The region for rejecting H_0 in a group-sequential clinical trial with the five planned analyses ($L = 5$), where the decision-making is based on DF-B. The hypothesis for the joint effect on both endpoints is tested at 2.5 % significance level. The critical boundaries for both endpoints are commonly determined by the OF, using the Lan–DeMets error-spending method, with equally spaced increments of information

statistics $Z_{14} = 3.5073$ for EP1 and $Z_{24} = 2.2294$ for EP2 at the fourth analysis, then H_0 is not rejected as Z_{14} is larger than the corresponding critical boundary of $c_{14}^E(2.5) = 2.2898$ but Z_{24} is not. At the final analysis, both H_{01} and H_{02} is tested again. If we observe $Z_{15} = 3.4946$ and $Z_{25} = 2.9732$, then H_0 is rejected as both Z_{15} and Z_{25} are larger than the corresponding critical boundary of $c_{15}^E(2.5) = c_{25}^E(2.5) = 2.0310$ simultaneously.

The power for the joint effect on both endpoints, corresponding to DF-B, is

$$1 - \beta = \Pr\left[\bigcup_{l=1}^{L}\{A_{1l} \cap A_{2l}\}\middle| H_1\right]. \tag{2.2}$$

Similarly as in the power based on DF-A, the power based on DF-B can be numerically assessed by using multivariate normal integrals. A detailed calculation is provided in Appendix A.

To illustrate the difference in the power for the joint effect on both endpoints between the DF-A and DF-B, Fig. 2.3 summarizes how the powers based on DF-A and DF-B behave with correlation ($\rho_T = \rho_C = \rho$), critical boundary combinations, and the number of planned analyses under a given sample size, in a group-sequential clinical trial with the two or four planned analyses ($L = 2$ or 4), assuming equal standardized mean differences $\Delta_1 = \Delta_2 = 0.2$. The hypothesis for the joint effect on both endpoints is tested at 2.5 % significance level. The given sample size (equally sized groups: $r_C = 1$) is 393 per intervention group has 80 % power to detect a standardized mean difference for each endpoint at 2.5 % significance level for a one-sided test. The three critical boundary combinations are considered: OF for both endpoints (OF-OF), Pocock-type boundary (PC) (Pocock 1977) for both endpoints (PC-PC), and OF for EP1 and PC for EP2 (OF-PC).

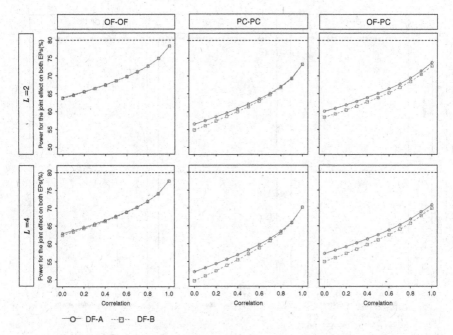

Fig. 2.3 Behavior of power for detecting a joint effect on both endpoints with correlation, critical boundary combinations, and the number of planned analyses under a given sample size, in a group-sequential clinical trial with the two or four planned analyses ($L = 2, 4$), assuming equal standardized mean differences $\Delta_1 = \Delta_2 = 0.2$, where the decision-making is based on DF-A or DF-B. The given sample size (equally sized groups) is 393 per intervention group has 80 % power to detect a standardized mean difference for each endpoint at 2.5 % significance level for a one-sided test. The hypothesis for the joint effect on both endpoints is tested at 2.5 % significance level. The critical boundary combinations are OF for both endpoints (OF-OF), and PC are for both endpoints (PC-PC) and OF for EP1 and PC for EP2 (OF-PC)

A range of correlation between the two endpoints considered in the evaluation is $\rho \geq 0$ since the correlation between the endpoints are usually non-negative as suggested in Offen et al. (2007).

The figure shows that the powers based on both DF-A and DF-B increase as the correlation approaches one in all of the three critical boundary combinations and the numbers of analyses. DF-A provides a slightly higher power than DF-B. In both of $L = 2$ and 4, the largest difference in the power between DF-A and DF-B is observed in PC-PC, and the smallest in OF-OF. However, the difference between DF-A and DF-B is smaller with higher correlation or smaller number of planned analyses in all of the three critical boundary combinations.

The testing procedure for co-primary endpoints is conservative. For example, in fixed-sample designs, if a zero correlation between the two endpoints is assumed and each endpoint is tested at 2.5 % significance level for a one-sided test, then the Type I error rate is 0.0625 % (=2.5 % × 2.5 %) (DF-A). As shown in Asakura

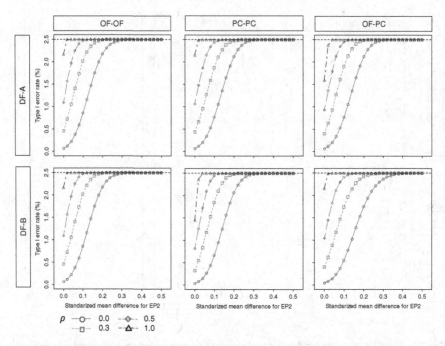

Fig. 2.4 Behavior of Type I error rate with correlation, critical boundary combinations, and standardized mean difference for EP2 in a group-sequential clinical trial with the two planned analyses ($L = 2$), assuming zero standardized mean difference for EP1 $\Delta_1 = 0$, where the decision-making is based on DF-A or DF-B. The hypothesis for the joint effect on both endpoints is tested at 2.5 % significance level. The three critical boundary combinations are OF for both endpoints (OF-OF), PC for both endpoints (PC-PC), OF for EP1 and PC for EP2 (OF-PC)

et al. (2014), the maximum overall Type I error rate associated with the rejection region of the null hypothesis increases as the correlation approaches one, but it is not larger than the prespecified significance level. Figure 2.4 summarizes how the overall Type I error rates based on DF-A and DF-B behave with correlation ($\rho_T = \rho_C = \rho$), critical boundary combinations, and standardized mean difference for EP2, in a group-sequential clinical trial with the two planned analyses ($L = 2$) and zero standardized mean difference for EP1, $\Delta_1 = 0.0$. The hypothesis for the joint effect on both endpoints is tested at 2.5 % significance level. The correlations are $\rho = 0.0$, 0.3, 0.5, and 1.0. The three critical boundary combinations are considered: OF for both endpoints (OF-OF), PC for both endpoints (PC-PC), and OF for EP1 and PC for EP2 (OF-PC). The figure shows that the Type I error rate for both decision-making frameworks increases as the correlation approaches one, but they are not larger than the prespecified significance level of 2.5 %, in all of the three critical boundary combinations, and DF-B is always slightly conservative than DF-A.

The above differences in power and the Type I error between DF-A and DF-B can be illustrated from the following two situations where the interim analysis result is inconsistent with the final analysis result even when the alternative hypothesis is true; that is, (i) EP1 is statistically significant at the interim, but not at the final analysis and similarly, and (ii) EP2 is statistically significant at the interim, but not at the final analysis. Thus, DF-B fails to reject the null hypothesis in both situations even if the alternative hypothesis is true, but DF-A is able to reject the null hypothesis in both situations. However, the likelihood of this scenario occurring is low and hence little practical difference in the power and sample size determinations based on DF-A and DF-B. However, DF-A offers the option of stopping measurement of an endpoint for which superiority has been demonstrated. Stopping measurement may be desirable if the endpoint is very invasive or expensive but may also introduce an operational challenge into the trial. For more details, see Asakura et al. (2014) and Hamasaki et al. (2015).

2.2.3 Sample Sizes

We describe two sample size concepts, i.e., the maximum sample size (MSS) and the average sample number (ASN) (i.e., expected sample size) based on the power (2.1) or (2.2). The MSS is the sample size required for the final analysis to achieve the desired power $1 - \beta$. The MSS is given by the smallest integer not less than n_L satisfying the power for a group-sequential strategy at the prespecified δ_k, σ_k, and ρ_T and ρ_C with Fisher's information time for the interim analyses, n_l/n_L ($l = 1, ..., L$).

To identify the value of n_L, an easy strategy is a grid search to gradually increase (or decrease) n_L until the power under n_L exceeds (or falls below) the desired power. The grid search often requires considerable computing time, especially with a larger number of endpoints, a larger number of planned analyses, or a small mean difference. To reduce the computing time, the Newton–Raphson algorithm in Sugimoto et al. (2012) or the basic linear interpolation algorithm in Hamasaki et al. (2013) may be utilized.

The ASN is the expected sample size under hypothetical reference values and provides information regarding the number of participants anticipated in a group-sequential clinical trial in order to reach a decision point. The ASN per intervention group is given by

$$\text{ASN} = \sum_{l=1}^{L-1} n_l P_l + n_L \left(1 - \sum_{l=1}^{L-1} P_l \right),$$

where $P_l = P_l(\delta_1, \delta_2, \sigma_1, \sigma_2, \rho_T, \rho_C)$ is the stopping probability (or exit probability) as defined by the likelihood of crossing the critical boundaries at the lth interim analysis assuming that the true values of the intervention's effect are (δ_1, δ_2).

Both MSS and ASN depend on the design parameters including the differences in means, the correlation structure among the endpoints, the selected critical boundary based on Lan–DeMets error-spending method, the number of planned analyses, and whether there are equally or unequally spaced increments of information. As shown in Hamasaki et al. (2015), our experience suggests that when considering more than two endpoints as co-primary in a group-sequential setting with more than five analyses, calculating the multivariate normal integrals often requires considerable computing time. A Monte Carlo simulation-based method provides an alternative but the number of replications for simulations should be carefully chosen to control simulation error in calculating the empirical power.

Figures 2.5 and 2.6 display how the reduction in MSS and ASN varies with the ratio of the two standardized mean differences (Δ_2/Δ_1), correlation ($\rho_T = \rho_C = \rho$),

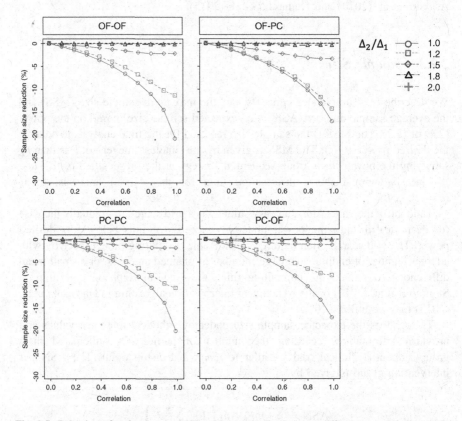

Fig. 2.5 Behavior of reduction in MSS with standardized mean difference, correlation, and critical boundary combination in a group-sequential clinical trial with the two planned analyses ($L = 2$), where the decision-making is based on DF-A. The sample size reduction is calculated as [MSS(ρ) – MSS(0)]/MSS(0), where MSS(ρ) is MSS calculated using ρ and MSS(0) is calculated using zero correlation. The sample size (equally sized groups) per intervention group is calculated to detect the joint effect on both endpoints with 80 % power at 2.5 % significance level for a one-sided test. The four critical boundary combinations are OF for both endpoints (OF-OF), PC for both endpoints (PC-PC), OF for EP1 and PC for EP2 (OF-PC), and PC for EP1 and OF for EP2 (PC-OF)

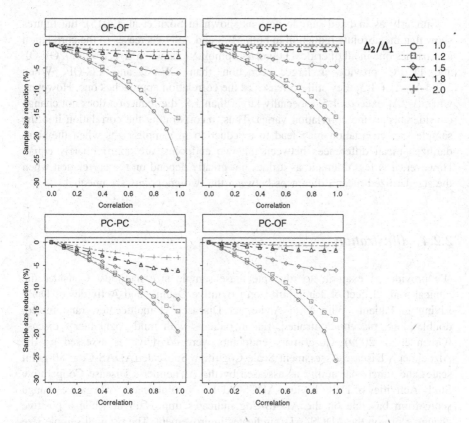

Fig. 2.6 Behavior of reduction in ASN with standardized mean difference, correlation, and critical boundary combination in a group-sequential clinical trial with the two planned analyses ($L = 2$), where the decision-making is based on DF-A. The reduction is calculated as $[MSS(\rho) - MSS(0)]/MSS(0)$, where $MSS(\rho)$ is MSS calculated using ρ and $MSS(0)$ is calculated using zero correlation. The sample size per intervention group (equally sized groups) is calculated to detect the joint effect on both endpoints with 80 % power at 2.5 % significance level for a one-sided test. The four critical boundary combinations are OF for both endpoints (OF-OF), PC for both endpoints (PC-PC), OF for EP1 and PC for EP2 (OF-PC), and PC for EP1 and OF for EP2 (PC-OF)

and critical boundary combinations in a group-sequential clinical trial with the two planned analyses ($L = 2$), where the decision-making is based on DF-A. The reduction is calculated as $[MSS(\rho) - MSS(0)]/MSS(0)$, where $MSS(\rho)$ is MSS calculated using ρ and $MSS(0)$ is calculated using zero correlation. The sample size per intervention group (equally sized groups: $r_C = 1$) is calculated to detect the joint effect on both endpoints with 80 % power at 2.5 % significance level for a one-sided test. The four critical boundary combinations are considered: OF for both endpoints (OF-OF), PC for both endpoints (PC-PC), OF for EP1 and PC for EP2 (OF-PC), and PC for EP1 and OF for EP2 (PC-OF).

Similarly as in fixed-sample designs shown in Sozu et al. (2015), the figures show that the absolute reduction in both MSS and ASN decreases as the correlation approaches one in all of critical boundary combinations when $\Delta_2/\Delta_1 = 1.0$. OF-OF and PC-PC provide a larger reduction than OF-PC and PC-OF. When $1.0 < \Delta_2/\Delta_1 < 1.5$, they still decreases as the correlation approaches one. However, when Δ_2/Δ_1 exceeds 1.5, especially larger than 1.8, the reduction does not change considerably as the correlation varies. Thus, incorporating the correlation into the sample size calculation may lead to a reduction in sample sizes when the standardized mean differences between the two endpoints are approximately equal. However, it is less dramatic as it does not greatly depend on the correlation when the standardized mean differences between the two endpoints are unequal.

2.2.4   Illustration

We provide an example to illustrate these sample size methods. Consider the clinical trial, "Effect of Tarenflurbil on Cognitive Decline and Activities of Daily Living in Patients With Mild Alzheimer Disease," a multicenter, randomized, double-blind, placebo-controlled trial in patients with mild Alzheimer's disease (Green et al. 2009). Co-primary endpoints were cognitive as assessed by the Alzheimer's Disease Assessment Scale Cognitive Subscale (ADAS-Cog: 80-point scale) and functional ability as assessed by the Alzheimer's Disease Cooperative Study Activities of Daily Living (ADCS–ADL: 78-point scale). A negative change score from baseline on the ADAS-Cog indicates improvement while a positive change score on the ADCS–ADL indicates improvement. The original sample size per intervention group (equally sized groups) of 800 patients provided 96 % power to detect the joint effect on the two primary endpoints, by using a one-sided test at 2.5 % significance level, with the standardized mean differences for both endpoints of $\Delta_1 = \Delta_2 = 0.2$. The correlation between the two endpoints was assumed to be zero in the calculation of the sample size although the two endpoints were expected to be correlated [for example, see Doraiswamy et al. (1997)].

Based on the selected parameters described in Green et al. (2009), i.e., $L = 1$ and $\rho_T = \rho_C = \rho = 0.0$, the sample size per intervention group is calculated as 804. As shown in Table 2.2, if four interims and one final analysis are planned (i.e., $L = 5$) based on DF-B, and conservatively assuming a zero correlation between the endpoints, then the MSS is 822 for OF-OF, 945 for PC-PC and 895 for OF-PC, and the ASN is 602 for OF-OF, 548 for PC-PC, and 608 for OF-PC. If the correlation is incorporated into the calculation when $\rho = 0.3$, 0.5, and 0.8, the MSS are 817, 809, and 782 for OF-OF; 939, 929, and 898 for PC-PC; and 890, 883, and 859 for OF-PC.

Table 2.1 MSS and ASN per intervention group (equally sized groups) for detecting the joint difference for ADAS-Cog ($\Delta_1 = 0.2$) and ADCS–ADL ($\Delta_2 = 0.2$), with the power of $1 - \beta = 96\%$ for detect the joint effect on both endpoints at 2.5 % significance level for one-sided test, based on DF-A

Correlation ρ	# of analyses L	OF-OF		PC-PC		OF-PC	
		MSS	ASN (H_1)	MSS	ASN (H_1)	MSS	ASN (H_1)
0.0	1	804		804		804	
	2	807	725	881	605	847	690
	3	813	645	911	570	867	647
	4	817	618	927	551	878	615
	5	821	601	937	540	886	600
0.3	1	799		799		799	
	2	801	702	875	591	841	672
	3	807	632	905	550	861	633
	4	812	602	921	530	873	602
	5	815	586	931	519	880	586
0.5	1	791		791		791	
	2	793	683	867	578	833	658
	3	799	619	896	534	854	622
	4	804	589	912	513	865	590
	5	807	572	922	502	873	574
0.8	1	764		764		764	
	2	767	643	839	548	809	631
	3	773	589	869	500	830	599
	4	777	557	884	478	841	566
	5	781	542	894	466	849	550

The three critical boundary combinations are OF for both endpoints (OF-OF), PC for both endpoints (PC-PC), and OF for EP1 and PC for EP2 (OF-PC). The ASN is calculated under H_1 ($\Delta_1 = \Delta_2 = 0.2$)

The ASN are 587, 574, and 542 for OF-OF; 525, 506, and 468 for PC-PC; and 593, 581, and 556 for OF-PC. When comparing DF-A (Table 2.1) to DF-B (Table 2.2), there are no major differences in MSS and ASN for all of the critical boundary combinations, although DF-A provides a slightly smaller MSS and ASN than DF-B, for PC-PC and OF-PC. The advantage and disadvantage of the decision-making frameworks are given in Sect. 2.5.

Figure 2.7 illustrates the probability of rejecting/not rejecting the null hypothesis under H_1 in a group-sequential clinical trial with the five planned analyses ($L = 5$), assuming the correlation $\rho = 0.0$ or 0.8, where the decision-making is based on DF-A. The figure shows that the method offers the possibility to stop a trial early if

Table 2.2 MSS and ASN per intervention group (equally sized groups) for detecting the joint difference for ADAS-Cog ($\Delta_1 = 0.2$) and ADCS–ADL ($\Delta_2 = 0.2$), with the power of $1 - \beta = 96$ % to detect the joint effect on both endpoints at 2.5 % significance level for one-sided test, based on DF-B

Correlation ρ	# of analyses L	OF-OF		PC-PC		OF-PC	
		MSS	ASN (H_1)	MSS	ASN (H_1)	MSS	ASN (H_1)
0.0	1	804		804		804	
	2	807	725	885	607	854	693
	3	814	646	917	574	875	653
	4	819	619	934	557	887	622
	5	822	602	945	548	895	608
0.3	1	799		799		799	
	2	802	702	880	593	849	676
	3	808	632	911	553	870	639
	4	813	603	928	535	882	608
	5	817	587	939	525	890	593
0.5	1	791		791		791	
	2	794	684	871	580	841	661
	3	800	620	902	537	863	628
	4	805	589	919	517	875	597
	5	809	574	929	506	883	581
0.8	1	764		764		764	
	2	767	643	841	549	818	635
	3	773	589	871	501	839	604
	4	778	558	887	480	851	571
	5	782	542	898	468	859	556

The three critical boundary combinations are considered: OF for both endpoints (OF-OF), PC for both endpoints (PC-PC), and OF for ADAS-Cog and PC for ADCS–ADL (OF-PC). The ASN is calculated under H_1 ($\Delta_1 = \Delta_2 = 0.2$)

evidence is overwhelming and thus offers potentially fewer patients than the fixed-sample designs. In the OF-OF and PC-OF testing procedure combinations, it is more difficult to reject the null hypothesis at the earliest analyses, but easier later on. On the other hand, in the PC-PC and OF-PC testing procedure combination, it is easier to reject the null hypothesis at the earliest analysis.

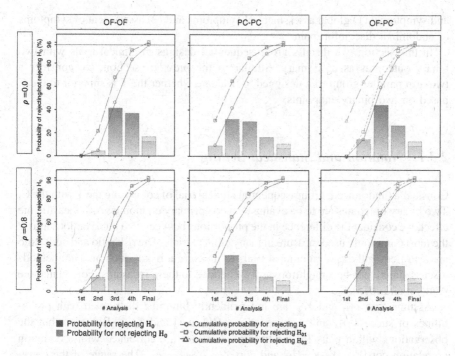

Fig. 2.7 The probability of rejecting/not rejecting the null hypothesis under H_1 in a group-sequential clinical trial with the five planned analyses ($L = 5$), where the decision-making is based on DF-A. The MSS are calculated to detect the joint effect for both endpoints with 96 % power at 2.5 % significance level for one-sided test, based on the assumption $\Delta_1 = \Delta_2 = 0.2$ from the tarenflurbil study. The critical boundaries are determined using the Lan–DeMets error-spending method with equally spaced increments of information. The three critical boundary combinations are OF for both endpoints (OF-OF), PC for both endpoints (PC-PC), and OF for ADAS-Cog and PC for ADCS–ADL (OF-PC)

2.3 Binary Outcomes

Clinical trials are often conducted with the objective of comparing a test intervention with that of a standard intervention based on several binary outcomes. For example, irritable bowel syndrome (IBS) is one of the most common gastrointestinal disorders and is characterized by symptoms of abdominal pain, discomfort, and altered bowel function (Grundmann and Yoon 2010; American College of Gastroenterology 2013). The comparison of the interventions to treat IBS is based on the proportions of participants with adequate relief of abdominal pain and discomfort, and improvements in urgency, stool frequency, and stool consistency. As described in Chap. 1, Food and Drug Administration (FDA) recommends the use of two endpoints for assessing IBS signs and symptoms: (1) pain intensity and (2) stool frequency (FDA 2013). The Committee for Medicinal Products for Human Use (CHMP) (2008) recommends the use of two endpoints for assessing IBS signs and symptoms: (1) global assessment of symptoms and (2) assessment of symptoms of abdominal discomfort/pain.

In this section, we discuss group-sequential designs in clinical trials with two binary outcomes as co-primary. Similar to the previous section, we consider a two-arm parallel-group trial designed to evaluate whether the T is superior to the C based on two binary endpoints.

2.3.1   Notation and Statistical Setting

Consider a randomized, group-sequential clinical trial of comparing the T with the C. Two binary outcomes are to be evaluated as co-primary endpoints. As a measure the effect, we consider the difference in the proportions between two interventions as it is the most commonly used measure in many clinical trials. The risk ratio and odds ratio are also frequently used in clinical trials to measure a risk reduction. The methods discussed here can be straightforwardly extended to these measures. For details, see Ando et al. (2015).

Assume that Y_{Tki} and Y_{Ckj} are independently binomial distributed with probabilities of success p_{Tk} and p_{Ck}, i.e., $Y_{Tki} \sim B(1, p_{Tk})$ and $Y_{Ckj} \sim B(1, p_{Ck})$, but the observations within pairs for the two interventions are correlated with a common correlation $\mathrm{corr}[Y_{T1i}, Y_{T2i}] = \rho_T$ and $\mathrm{corr}[Y_{C1j}, Y_{C2j}] = \rho_C$. The range of the correlations ρ_T and ρ_C are restricted, depending on the marginal probabilities (Prentice 1988; Le Cessie and van Houwelingen 1994). Let (δ_1, δ_2) denote the differences in proportions for the T and the C, respectively, where $\delta_k = p_{Tk} - p_{Ck}$ $(k = 1, 2)$. Suppose that positive values of (δ_1, δ_2) represent the test intervention's benefit. We now have the two observed differences in proportions at the lth analysis, i.e., $(\hat{\delta}_1, \hat{\delta}_2)$, where $\hat{\delta}_{kl} = \hat{p}_{Tkl} - \hat{p}_{Ckl}$ with $\hat{p}_{Tkl} = Y_{Tkl}/n_l$ and $\hat{p}_{Ckl} = Y_{Ckl}/r_C n_l$, and $Y_{Tkl} = \sum_{i=1}^{n_l} Y_{T1i}$ and $Y_{Ckl} = \sum_{j=1}^{r_C n_l} Y_{Ckj}$ denote the number of success under the T and the C. It follows that $Y_{Tkl} \sim B(n_l, p_{Tk})$ and $Y_{Ckl} \sim B(r_C n_l, p_{Ck})$.

We are interested in conducting a hypothesis test to evaluate whether the T is superior to the C, i.e., the null hypothesis H_0: $\delta_1 \leq 0$ or $\delta_2 \leq 0$ versus the alternative hypothesis H_1: $\delta_1 > 0$ and $\delta_2 > 0$. Let (Z_{1l}, Z_{2l}) be the Z-score statistics for testing the hypotheses at the lth analysis, given by

$$Z_{kl} = \frac{\hat{p}_{Tkl} - \hat{p}_{Ckl}}{\sqrt{\hat{\bar{p}}_{kl}\hat{\bar{q}}_{kl}(r_C + 1/r_C)/n_l}},$$

where $\hat{\bar{p}}_{kl} = (\hat{p}_{Tkl} + r_C \hat{p}_{Ckl})/(1 + r_C)$ and $\hat{\bar{q}}_{kl} = 1 - \hat{\bar{p}}_{kl}$. For large samples, each Z_{kl} is approximately normally distributed [e.g., see Fleiss et al. (2003)]. Thus, the two test statistics at lth analysis (Z_{1l}, Z_{2l}) is approximately bivariate normally distributed with the correlation

$$\mathrm{corr}[Z_{1l}, Z_{2l}] = \rho_Z = \frac{r_C\rho_T\sqrt{p_{T1}q_{T1}p_{T2}q_{T2}} + \rho_C\sqrt{p_{C1}q_{C1}p_{C2}q_{C2}}}{\sqrt{r_Cp_{T1}q_{T1} + p_{C1}q_{C1}}\sqrt{r_Cp_{T2}q_{T2} + p_{C2}q_{C2}}},$$

$q_{Tk} = 1 - p_{Tk}$ and $q_{Ck} = 1 - p_{Ck}$. Furthermore, the joint distribution of $(Z_{11}, Z_{21}, \ldots, Z_{1l}, Z_{2l}, \ldots, Z_{1L}, Z_{2L})$ is approximately $2L$ multivariate normal with their correlations given by $\mathrm{corr}[Z_{1l'}, Z_{1l}] = \mathrm{corr}[Z_{2l'}, Z_{2l}] = \sqrt{n_{l'}/n_l}$ and $\mathrm{corr}[Z_{1l'}, Z_{2l}] = \mathrm{corr}[Z_{1l}, Z_{2l'}] = \rho_Z\sqrt{n_{l'}/n_l}$, where $1 \leq l' \leq l \leq L$. Similarly as discussed in Sect. 2.2, we can calculate the power, Type I error rate, and sample sizes based on the two decision-making frameworks associated with hypothesis testing, i.e., DF-A and DF-B.

The method is based on the normal approximation which works well in most situations (Asakura et al. 2015). However, it may not work well in the occurrence of extremely small event rates or small sample sizes as the joint distribution is not fully specified in the first- and second-order moments. In such situations, Monte Carlo simulation-based method or more direct methods may be more appropriate although this occurs at the expense of considerable computational resources. For more direct methods for multiple co-primary endpoints in fixed-sample designs including Fisher's exact test, see Sozu et al. (2010, 2015).

2.3.2 Illustration

We provide an example to illustrate these sample size methods. Consider the double-blind, randomized, parallel-group, placebo-controlled trial evaluating lactobacilli and bifidobacteria in the prevention of antibiotic-associated diarrhea in older people admitted to hospital (the PLACIDE study) (Allen et al. 2012, 2013). The study was designed to demonstrate that the administration of a probiotic comprising two strains of lactobacilli and two strains of bifidobacteria alongside antibiotic treatment prevents antibiotic-associated diarrhea. The co-primary outcomes were: (EP1) the occurrence of antibiotic-associated diarrhea (AAD) within 8 weeks and (EP2) the occurrence of C *difficile* diarrhea (CDD) within 12 weeks of recruitment.

The original sample size per intervention group (equally sized groups) of 1239 participants provided 80 % power to detect a 50 % reduction in CDD in the probiotic group compared with the placebo group, by using a two-sided Fisher's exact test at 5 % significance level, assuming CDD frequencies of 4 % in placebo group and 2 % in probiotic group. Although Cochran's condition seems to be hold for this setting, the normal approximation method was not used for the sample size calculation and the sample size was conservatively calculated. This sample size would provide a power of more than 99 % to detect a 50 % reduction in AAD, by using a two-sided Fisher's exact test at 5 % significance level, assuming AAD frequencies of 20 % in placebo group and 10 % in probiotic group as the normal approximation. The correlation between the two outcomes was not incorporated into the original sample size calculation.

Tables 2.3 and 2.4 display the MSS and ASN per intervention group (equally sized groups: $r_C = 1$) based on DF-A and DF-B. The sample size was derived using an alternative hypothesis of differences in proportions for AAD ($p_{T1} = 0.2$ and $p_{C1} = 0.4$) and CDD ($p_{T2} = 0.02$ and $p_{C2} = 0.04$) with 80 % power at 2.5 % significance level for one-sided test, using the normal approximation method where $\rho = \rho_T = \rho_C = 0.0, 0.3, 0.5$, and 0.8; $L = 2, 3, 4$, and 5. The critical boundaries are determined by using the Lan–DeMets error-spending method, with equally spaced increments of information. The critical boundary combinations are OF for both endpoints (OF-OF), PC for both endpoints (PC-PC), OF for AAD and PC for CDD (OF-PC), and PC for AAD and OF for CDD (PC-OF).

Based on the selected parameters described in Allen et al. (2012), i.e., $L = 1$ and $\rho = 0.0$, the sample size per intervention group (equally sized groups) is calculated as 1141. If four interims and one final analysis are planned (i.e., $L = 5$) based on DF-A, and conservatively assuming a zero correlation between the endpoints, then

Table 2.3 MSS and ASN per intervention group (equally sized groups) for detecting the joint difference for AAD ($p_{T1} = 0.2$ and $p_{C1} = 0.4$) and CDD ($p_{T2} = 0.02$ and $p_{C2} = 0.04$), with 80 % power at 2.5 % significance level for a one-sided test, where the decision-making is based on DF-A

Correlation ρ	# of analyses L	OF-OF		PC-PC		OF-PC		PC-OF	
		MSS	ASN (H_1)	MSS	ASN (H_1)	MSS	ASN (H_1)	MSS	ASN (H_1)
0.0	2	1146	1056	1282	977	1282	982	1146	1053
	3	1156	991	1337	941	1337	981	1156	989
	4	1164	960	1366	925	1366	972	1164	958
	5	1170	943	1385	918	1385	956	1170	941
0.3	2	1146	1056	1282	977	1282	982	1146	1053
	3	1156	991	1337	941	1337	981	1156	989
	4	1164	960	1366	925	1366	972	1164	958
	5	1170	943	1385	918	1385	956	1170	941
0.5	2	1146	1056	1282	977	1282	982	1146	1053
	3	1156	991	1337	941	1337	981	1156	989
	4	1164	960	1366	925	1366	972	1164	958
	5	1170	943	1385	918	1385	956	1170	941
0.8	2	1146	1056	1282	977	1282	982	1146	1053
	3	1156	991	1337	941	1337	981	1156	989
	4	1164	960	1366	925	1366	972	1164	958
	5	1170	943	1385	918	1385	956	1170	941

The critical boundaries are determined by using the Lan–DeMets error-spending method, with equally spaced increments of information. The critical boundary combinations are OF for both endpoints (OF-OF), PC for both endpoints (PC-PC), OF for AAD and PC for CDD (OF-PC), and PC for AAD and OF for CDD (PC-OF). The ASN is calculated under H_1 ($p_{T1} = 0.2$ and $p_{C1} = 0.4$, and $p_{T2} = 0.02$ and $p_{C2} = 0.04$)

Table 2.4 MSS and ASN per intervention group (equally sized groups) for detecting the joint difference for AAD ($p_{T1} = 0.2$ and $p_{C1} = 0.4$) and CDD ($p_{T2} = 0.02$ and $p_{C2} = 0.04$), with 80 % at power at 2.5 % significance level for a one-sided test, where the decision-making is based on DF-B

Correlation ρ	# of analyses L	OF-OF MSS	OF-OF ASN (H_1)	PC-PC MSS	PC-PC ASN (H_1)	OF-PC MSS	OF-PC ASN (H_1)	PC-OF MSS	PC-OF ASN (H_1)
0.0	2	1146	1056	1282	977	1283	983	1146	1053
	3	1156	991	1337	941	1346	989	1156	989
	4	1164	960	1368	928	1380	989	1164	958
	5	1170	944	1387	921	1399	976	1170	941
0.3	2	1146	1055	1282	977	1283	982	1146	1053
	3	1156	991	1337	940	1346	985	1156	989
	4	1164	959	1367	926	1380	987	1164	958
	5	1170	943	1387	920	1398	973	1170	941
0.5	2	1146	1055	1282	977	1283	982	1146	1053
	3	1156	991	1337	940	1346	985	1156	989
	4	1164	959	1367	926	1380	987	1164	958
	5	1170	943	1387	920	1398	973	1170	941
0.8	2	1146	1055	1282	977	1283	982	1146	1053
	3	1156	991	1337	940	1346	985	1156	989
	4	1164	959	1367	926	1380	987	1164	958
	5	1170	943	1387	920	1398	973	1170	941

The critical boundaries are determined by using the Lan–DeMets error-spending method, with equally spaced increments of information. The critical boundary combinations are OF for both endpoints (OF-OF), PC for both endpoints (PC-PC), OF for AAD and PC for CDD (OF-PC), and PC for AAD and OF for CDD (PC-OF). The ASN is calculated under H_1 ($p_{T1} = 0.2$ and $p_{C1} = 0.4$, and $p_{T2} = 0.02$ and $p_{C2} = 0.04$)

the MSS is 1170 for OF-OF, 1387 for PC-PC, 1399 for OF-PC, and 1170 for PC-OF, and the ASN is 944 for OF-OF, 921 for PC-PC, 976 for OF-PC, and 941 for PC-OF. On the other hand, even if the correlation is incorporated into the calculation, the MSS and ASN do not change as the correlation varies. This means that when one standardized difference in proportions is relatively larger than the other, i.e., $\delta_1 > \delta_2$ (or $\delta_1 < \delta_2$) with $p_{C1} \neq p_{C2}$, then there is little benefit in incorporating the correlation into sample size calculation.

When comparing DF-A (Table 2.3) to DF-B (Table 2.4), there are no major differences in MSS and ASN for all of the testing procedure combinations, although DF-A provides a slightly smaller MSS and ASN than DF-B: for DF-B, the MSS is 1170 for OF-OF, 1387 for PC-PC, 1399 for OF-PC, and 1170 for PC-OF, and the ASN is 944 for OF-OF, 921 for PC-PC, 976 for OF-PC, and 941 for PC-OF when assuming a zero correlation.

2.4 Practical Issues

Two important decisions must be made when constructing efficient group-sequential strategies in clinical trials with multiple co-primary endpoints. The first decision is the choice of the critical boundary based on an error-spending method for each endpoint. If the trial was designed to detect effects on at least one endpoint with a prespecified ordering of endpoints, then the selection of different boundaries for each endpoint (i.e., the OF for the primary endpoint and the PC for the secondary endpoint) can provide a higher power than using the same critical boundary for both endpoints (Glimm et al. 2010; Tamhane et al. 2010). However, as shown in Asakura et al. (2014), the selection of a different critical boundary has a minimal effect on the overall power and ASN. In both decision-making frameworks, regardless of equal or unequal standardized mean difference among the endpoints, the largest power is obtained from the OF for all of the endpoints, and the lowest is the PC for all of the endpoints. Regarding the ASN, the smallest is provided by the PC for all of the endpoints while the largest is provided by the OF. One possible scenario for selecting a different boundary is when one endpoint is invasive and stopping measurement of the endpoint is desirable as soon as possible, i.e., once the superiority for the endpoint has been demonstrated.

Table 2.5 illustrates the average observation number (AON) per intervention group (equally sized groups) for each endpoint based on the decision-making frameworks DF-A under a given MSS in clinical trials with two co-primary endpoints, EP1 and EP2, when their standardized mean differences are $(\Delta_1, \Delta_2) = (0.2, 0.2)$ and $(0.2, 0.3)$. The AON is the expected sample size for each endpoint

Table 2.5 The AON per intervention group for each endpoint based on the decision-making framework DF-A under a given MSS in clinical trials with two co-primary endpoints, EP1 and EP2, when their standardized mean differences are $(\Delta_1, \Delta_2) = (0.2, 0.2)$ and $(0.2, 0.3)$

Standardized mean difference	Sample sizes		Critical boundary combination			
			OF-OF	PC-PC	OF-PC	PC-OF
(0.2, 0.2)	AON (H_{1k})	EP1	403	454	474	490
		EP2	403	454	390	474
		MSS	574	518	547	547
	ASN (H_1)		472	502	505	505
(0.2, 0.3)	AON (H_{1k})	EP1	259	298	316	243
		EP2	341	368	339	373
		MSS	450	403	446	408
	ASN (H_1)		357	385	384	380

The MSS per intervention group (equally sized groups) is calculated to detect the joint effect for two endpoints with 80 % power at 2.5 % significance level for a one-sided test, where one interim and one final analysis are to be performed. The critical boundaries are determined by using the Lan–DeMets error-spending method, with equally spaced increments of information. The critical boundary combinations are OF for both endpoints (OF-OF), PC for both endpoints (PC-PC), OF for AAD and PC for CDD (OF-PC), and PC for AAD and OF for CDD (PC-OF). The ASN is calculated under H_1 ($\Delta_1 = \Delta_2 = 0.2$). AON is calculated under H_{1k} with the calculated MSS and it is calculated under the hypothetical reference values and provides information on the number of observations anticipated in a group-sequential clinical trial in order to reach a decision point for each endpoint. The AON is calculated under H_{1k} with the calculated MSS. The MSS per intervention group (equally sized groups) is calculated to detect the joint effect for two endpoints with 80 % power at 2.5 % significance level for a one-sided test, where one interim and one final analysis are to be performed. The critical boundaries are determined by the combinations of the OF and the PC, using the Lan–DeMets error-spending method with equally spaced increments of information; if EP1 is an invasive endpoint, then the critical boundary combination of the PC for EP1 and the OF for EP2 provides the smallest AON for EP1 in all of the standardized mean difference combinations.

Another practical decision is the selection of the correlations in the power evaluation and sample size calculation, i.e., whether the observed correlation from external or pilot data should be utilized. As shown in Sect. 2.2.3, when the standardized mean differences for the endpoints are unequal, the advantage of incorporating the correlation into sample size calculation is less dramatic as the required sample size is primarily determined by the smaller standardized mean difference and does not greatly depend on the correlation. In this situation, the sample size equation for multiple co-primary continuous endpoints can be simplified using the equation for a single endpoint. When the standardized mean differences among endpoints are approximately equal, one conservative approach is to assume that the correlations are zero even if nonzero correlations are expected. Group-sequential designs discussed in this chapter offer the possibility of reducing the sample size compared to fixed-sample designs even if zero correlation is assumed at the design stage.

Table 2.6 summarizes MSS and ASN per intervention group in clinical trials with two co-primary endpoints. The MSS per intervention group (equally sized

Table 2.6 MSS and ASN per intervention group in clinical trials with two co-primary endpoints

Decision-making framework	# of analyses L	MSS	ASN (H_1)			
			0.0	0.3	0.5	0.8
DF-A	2	518	502	494	488	475
	3	522	470	461	455	442
	4	525	457	447	440	426
	5	528	449	440	432	418
DF-B	2	518	502	494	488	475
	3	523	471	462	455	443
	4	528	459	449	442	428
	5	530	451	441	434	419

The MSS per intervention group (equally sized groups) is calculated to detect the joint effect for two endpoints ($\Delta_1 = \Delta_2 = 0.2$) with 80 % power at 2.5 % significance level for a one-sided test, where the correlation between the two endpoints is assumed to be zero, i.e., $\rho_T = \rho_C = \rho = 0.0$ and the critical boundaries are determined by OF, using the Lan–DeMets error-spending method with equally spaced increments of information. The ASN is calculated under H_1 ($\Delta_1 = \Delta_2 = 0.2$) with $\rho = 0.0, 0.3, 0.5,$ and 0.8

groups) is calculated to detect the joint effect for two endpoints with 80 % power at 2.5 % significance level for a one-sided test, where the correlation between the two endpoints is assumed to be zero, i.e., $\rho_T = \rho_C = \rho = 0.0$ and the critical boundaries are determined by the ·OF, using the Lan–DeMets error-spending method with equally spaced increments of information. The ASN is calculated under H_1 ($\Delta_1 = \Delta_2 = 0.2$) and $\rho = 0.0, 0.3, 0.5,$ and 0.8. For example, when considering a clinical trial with two co-primary endpoints, 516, 503, 490, 458 participants per intervention group are required to detect a joint effect of equal standardized mean difference $\Delta_1 = \Delta_2 = 0.2$ with 80 % power at 2.5 % significance level for a one-sided test in a fixed-sample design, if the correlation between two endpoints is $\rho = 0.0, 0.3, 0.5,$ and 0.8. In a group-sequential design based on DF-B, assuming zero correlation between the two endpoints, the MSS are 518, 523, 528, and 530 corresponding to the number of planned analyses $L = 2, 3, 4,$ and 5. The critical boundaries for both endpoints are determined by OF, using the Lan–DeMets error-spending method with equally spaced increments of information. Under these MSS, the ASN are 488, 455, 442, and 434. The ASN are approximately equal or smaller than the fixed-sample designs, depending on the number of planned analyses. Our experience suggests that when standardized mean differences are unequal among the endpoints, the power is not increased with higher correlations. With unequal standardized mean differences, incorporating the correlation into the sample size calculation at the planning stage may have less of an advantage because the sample size is determined by the smaller standardized mean difference.

2.5   Summary

The determination of sample size and the evaluation of power are fundamental and critical elements in the design of a clinical trial. If a sample size is too small, then important effects may not be detected, while a sample size that is too large is wasteful of resources and unethically puts more participants at risk than necessary. Recently, many clinical trials are designed with more than one endpoint considered as co-primary. As with trials involving a single primary endpoint, designing such trials to include interim analyses (i.e., with repeated testing) may provide efficiencies by detecting trends prior to planned completion of the trial. It may also be prudent to evaluate design assumptions at the interim and potentially make design adjustments (i.e., sample size recalculation) if design assumptions were dramatically inaccurate. However, such design complexities create challenges in the evaluation of power and the calculation of sample size during trial design.

In this chapter, we discuss group-sequential designs with two co-primary endpoints, where both endpoints are continuous or both are binary. We derive the power and sample size methods under two decision-making frameworks: (1) designing the trial to detect superiority for the two endpoints at any interim time-point (i.e., not necessarily simultaneously) (DF-A) and (2) designing the trial to detect the test intervention's superiority for the two endpoints simultaneously (i.e., at the same

Table 2.7 Advantages and disadvantages of the two decision-making frameworks in clinical trials with multiple co-primary endpoints

Decision-making framework	Advantages	Disadvantages
DF-A	• Controls the Type I error rate adequately • Flexible to allow the option of selecting different timings for interim analyses among the endpoints; this is useful when designing clinical trials with the endpoints requiring different information times such as progression-free survival and overall survival • Possible to stop measuring an endpoint for which superiority has been demonstrated—this is desirable if the endpoint is very invasive or expensive (e.g., data from a liver biopsy or gastro-fiberscope, or data from expensive imaging)	• Conservative as the rejection region of the null hypothesis becomes more restricted as the number of endpoints increases • Difficult to maintain the integrity and validity of clinical trial if stopping measurement of an endpoint for which superiority has been demonstrated
DF-B	• Controls the Type I error rate adequately • Makes the decision-making simple and easy to use in practice	• Conservative as the rejection region of the null hypothesis becomes more restricted as the number of endpoints increases • Cannot stop measuring an endpoint for which superiority has been demonstrated • Provides the lowest power and largest sample sizes among the decision-making frameworks

interim time-point of the trial) (DF-B). The latter is simpler while the former is more flexible and may be useful when the endpoint is very invasive or expensive, as it allows for stopping the measurement of any endpoint upon which superiority has been demonstrated. We summarize advantages and disadvantages of the two decision-making frameworks in clinical trials with multiple co-primary endpoints in Table 2.7. For other decision-making frameworks, see Hamasaki et al. (2015).

References

Allen SJ, Wareham K, Bradley C, Harris W, Dhar A, Brown H, Foden A, Cheung WY, Gravenor MB, Plummer S, Phillips CJ, Mack D (2012) A multicentre randomised controlled trial evaluating lactobacilli and bifidobacteria in the prevention of antibiotic-associated diarrhoea in older people admitted to hospital: the PLACIDE study protocol. BMC Infect Dis 12:108

Allen SJ, Wareham K, Wang D, Bradley C, Hutchings H, Harris W, Dhar A, Brown H, Foden A, Gravenor MB, Mack D (2013) Lactobacilli and bifidobacteria in the prevention of antibiotic-associated diarrhoea and Clostridium difficile diarrhoea in older inpatients (PLACIDE): a randomised, double-blind, placebo-controlled, multicentre trial. Lancet 382:1249–1257

American College of Gastroenterology Website (2013) Understanding irritable bowel syndrome. www.patients.gi.org/gi-health-and-disease/understanding-irritable-bowel-syndromeleavingsiteicon. Accessed 25 Nov 2015

Ando Y, Hamasaki T, Evans SR, Asakura K, Sugimoto T, Sozu T, Ohno Y (2015) Sample size considerations in clinical trials when comparing two interventions using multiple co-primary binary relative risk contrasts. Stat Biopharm Res 7:81–89

Asakura K, Hamasaki T, Sugimoto T, Hayashi K, Evans SR, Sozu T (2014) Sample size determination in group-sequential clinical trials with two co-primary endpoints. Stat Med 33:2897–2913

Asakura K, Hamasaki T, Evans SR, Sugimoto T, Sozu T (2015) Group-sequential designs when considering two binary outcomes as co-primary endpoints. In: Chen Z, Liu A, Qu Y, Tang L, Ting N, Tsong Y (eds) Applied statistics in biomedicine and clinical trials design (Chap. 14). Springer International Publishing, Cham, pp 235–262

Berger RL (1982) Multiparameter hypothesis testing and acceptance sampling. Technometrics 24:295–300

Cheng Y, Ray S, Chang M, Menon S (2014) Statistical monitoring of clinical trials with multiple co-primary endpoints using multivariate B-value. Stat Biopharm Res 6:241–250

Committee for Medicinal Products for Human Use (2008) Guideline on medicinal products for the treatment Alzheimer's disease and Other dementias (CPMP/EWP/553/95 Rev.1). European Medicines Agency, London, UK. Available at: http://www.ema.europa.eu/docs/en_GB/document_library/Scientific_guideline/2009/09/WC500003562.pdf. Accessed 25 Nov 2015

Cook RJ, Farewell VT (1994) Guideline for monitoring efficacy and toxicity responses in clinical trials. Biometrics 50:1146–1162

Doraiswamy PM, Bieber F, Kaiser L, Krishnan KR, Reuning-Scherer J, Gulanski B (1997) The Alzheimer's disease assessment scale: patterns and predictors of baseline cognitive performance in multicenter Alzheimer's disease trials. Neurol 48:1511–1517

Fleiss JL, Levin B, Paik MC (2003) Statistical methods for rates and proportions, 3rd edn. Wiley, Hoboken

Food and Drug Administration (2013) Guidance for industry. Alzheimer's disease: developing drugs for the treatment of early stage disease. Center for Drug Evaluation and Research, Food and Drug Administration, Rockville, MD, USA. Available at: http://www.fda.gov/ucm/groups/fdagov-public/@fdagov-drugs-gen/documents/document/ucm338287.pdf. Accessed 25 Nov 2015

Glimm E, Maurer W, Bretz F (2010) Hierarchical testing of multiple endpoints in group-sequential trials. Stat Med 29:219–228

Green R et al (2009) Effect of tarenflurbil on cognitive decline and activities of daily living in patients with mild Alzheimer disease: a randomized controlled trial. J Am Med Assoc 302:2557–2564

Grundmann O, Yoon SL (2010) Irritable bowel syndrome: epidemiology, diagnosis, and treatment: an update for health-care practitioners. J Gastroenterol and Hepatol 25:691–699

Hamasaki T, Sugimoto T, Evans SR, Sozu T (2013) Sample size determination for clinical trials with co-primary outcomes: exponential event times. Pharm Stat 12:28–34

Hamasaki T, Asakura K, Evans SR, Sugimoto T, Sozu T (2015) Group sequential strategies for clinical trials with multiple co-primary endpoints. Stat Biopharm Res 7:36–54

Hung HMJ, Wang SJ (2009) Some controversial multiple testing problems in regulatory applications. J Biopharm Stat 19:1–11

Jennison C, Turnbull BW (1993) Group sequential tests for bivariate response: interim analyses of clinical trials with both efficacy and safety. Biometrics 49:741–752

Lan KKG, DeMets DL (1983) Discrete sequential boundaries for clinical trials. Biometrika 70:659–663

Le Cessie S, van Houwelingen JC (1994) Logistic regression for correlated binary data. Appl Stat 43:95–108

O'Brien PC, Fleming TR (1979) A multiple testing procedure for clinical trials. Biometrics 35:549–556

Offen W et al (2007) Multiple co-primary endpoints: medical and statistical solutions. Drug Inf J 41:31–46

Pocock SJ (1977) Group sequential methods in the design and analysis of clinical trials. Biometrika 64:191–199

Prentice RL (1988) Correlated binary regression with covariates specific to each binary observarion. Biometrics 44:1033–1048

Sozu T, Sugimoto T, Hamasaki T (2010) Sample size determination in clinical trials with multiple co-primary binary endpoints. Stat Med 29:2169–2179

Sozu T, Sugimoto T, Hamasaki T (2011) Sample size determination in superiority clinical trials with multiple co-primary correlated endpoints. J Biopharm Stat 21:1–19

Sozu T, Sugimoto T, Hamasaki T, Evans SR (2015) Sample size determination in clinical trials with multiple primary endpoints. Springer International Press, Cham

Sugimoto T, Sozu T, Hamasaki T (2012) A convenient formula for sample size calculations in clinical trials with multiple co-primary continuous endpoints. Pharm Stat 11:118–128

Tamhane AC, Mehta CR, Liu L (2010) Testing a primary and secondary endpoint in a group sequential design. Biometrics 66:1174–1184

Chapter 3
Sample Size Recalculation in Clinical Trials with Two Co-primary Endpoints

Abstract Clinical trial design requires assumptions. Prior data often serve as the basis for these assumptions. However, prior data may be limited or an inaccurate indication of future data. This may result in trials that are over-/under-powered. Interim analyses provide opportunities to evaluate the accuracy of the design assumptions and potentially make design adjustments if the assumptions are markedly inaccurate. We discuss sample size recalculation based on the observed intervention's effects during interim analyses with a focus on the control of statistical error rates.

Keywords Conditional power · Cui–Hung–Wang statistics · Sample size recalculation · Type I error

3.1 Sample Size Recalculation

Clinical trials are designed based on assumptions often constructed based on prior data. However, prior data may be limited or an inaccurate indication of future data, resulting in trials that are over-/under-powered. Interim analyses provide opportunities to evaluate the accuracy of the design assumptions and potentially make design adjustments (i.e., to the sample size) if the assumptions were markedly inaccurate. For example, the tarenflurbil trial (Green et al. 2009) mentioned in Chap. 2 failed to demonstrate a beneficial effect of tarenflurbil on both the Alzheimer's Disease Assessment Scale Cognitive Subscale (ADAS-Cog) and the Alzheimer's Disease Cooperative Study Activities of Daily Living (ADCS–ADL). The observed treatment effects were smaller than the assumed effects. Group-sequential designs allow for early stopping when there is sufficient statistical evidence that the two treatments are different. However, more modern adaptive designs may also allow for increases in the sample size if effects are smaller than assumed. Such adjustments must be conducted carefully for several reasons. Challenges include the following:

© The Author(s) 2016
T. Hamasaki et al., *Group-Sequential Clinical Trials with Multiple Co-Objectives*,
JSS Research Series in Statistics, DOI 10.1007/978-4-431-55900-9_3

- Maintaining control of statistical error rates,
- Developing a plan to make sure that treatment effects cannot be inferred via back-calculation of a resulting change in the sample size,
- Consideration of the clinical relevance of the treatment effects, and
- Practical concerns such as an increase in cost and the challenge of accruing more trial participants.

In this chapter, we discuss sample size recalculation based on the observed intervention's effects at an interim analysis with a focus on the control of statistical error rates.

3.2 Test Statistics and Conditional Power

Using the notation defined in Chap. 2, we consider a two-arm parallel-group trial designed to evaluate if a test intervention (T) is superior to a control (C) based on two continuous outcomes EP1 and EP2 ($K = 2$) as co-primary endpoints. Suppose that the groups are equally sized and a maximum of L analyses is planned, where the same number of planned analyses with the same information space is selected for both endpoints. Let n_l be the cumulative number of participants on the T and the C at the lth analysis ($l = 1, \ldots, L$), respectively. Hence, up to n_L participants are recruited and randomly assigned to the T and the C, respectively. Then, there are n_L paired outcomes (Y_{T1i}, Y_{T2i}) ($i = 1, \ldots, n_L$) for the T and n_L paired outcomes (Y_{C1j}, Y_{C2j}) ($j = 1, \ldots, n_L$) for the C. Assume that (Y_{T1i}, Y_{T2i}) and (Y_{C1j}, Y_{C2j}) are independently bivariate distributed with mean $E[Y_{Tki}] = \mu_{Tk}$ and $E[Y_{Ckj}] = \mu_{Ck}$, variances $\mathrm{var}[Y_{Tki}] = \sigma_{Tk}^2$ and $\mathrm{var}[Y_{Ckj}] = \sigma_{Ck}^2$, and correlation $\mathrm{corr}[Y_{T1i}, Y_{T2i}] = \rho_T$ and $\mathrm{corr}[Y_{C1j}, Y_{C2j}] = \rho_C$, respectively ($k = 1, 2$). For simplicity, the variances are assumed to be known and common, i.e., $\sigma_{Tk}^2 = \sigma_{Ck}^2 = \sigma_k^2$.

Let $\delta_k = \mu_{Tk} - \mu_{Ck}$ and $\Delta_k = \delta_k / \sigma_k$ denote the mean differences and standardized mean differences for the T and the C, respectively ($k = 1, 2$). Suppose that positive values of δ_k represent the test intervention's benefit. There is an interest in testing $H_0 : H_{01} \cup H_{02}$ versus $H_1 : H_{11} \cap H_{12}$ at the α level within the context of group-sequential designs, where $H_{0k}{:}\delta_k \leq 0$ and $H_{1k}{:}\delta_k > 0$ with $\delta_k = \mu_{Tk} - \mu_{Ck}$.

Consider that the maximum sample size (MSS) is recalculated to n_L' based on the interim data at the Sth analysis. Suppose that n_L' is subject to $n_R < n_L' < \lambda n_L$, where λ is a prespecified constant for the maximum allowable sample size. For simplicity, assume a common correlation between the treatment groups, i.e., $\rho_T = \rho_C = \rho$. Without loss of generality, let $(\tilde{\Delta}_1, \tilde{\Delta}_2)$ and let (Δ_1^*, Δ_2^*) be the standardized mean differences used for planned sample size and for recalculated sample size, respectively.

Here, we consider the Cui–Hung–Wang (CHW) statistics (Cui et al. 1999) for sample size recalculation in group-sequential designs with two co-primary endpoints to preserve the overall Type I error rate at a prespecified significance level even when the sample size is increased and conventional test statistics are used. Using the notation defined in Chap. 2, if the CHW statistics are

$$
Z'_{km} = \sqrt{\frac{n_S}{n_m}} Z_{kS} + \sqrt{\frac{n_m - n_S}{n_m}} \frac{\sum_{i=n_S+1}^{n'_m} Y_{Tki} - \sum_{j=n_S+1}^{n'_m} Y_{Ckj}}{\sqrt{2(n'_m - n_S)}}
$$

where $n'_m = (n_m - n_S)(n'_L - n_S)/(n_L - n_S) + n_S (k = 1, 2; \ S = 1, \ldots, L-1;$ and $m = S+1, \ldots, L)$, and Z_{kS} is the test statistic at the Sth analysis for endpoint k $(k = 1, 2)$, which is given by

$$
Z_{kS} = \frac{\overline{Y}_{TkS} - \overline{Y}_{CkS}}{\sigma_k \sqrt{2/n_S}},
$$

where $\overline{Y}_{TkS}$ and $\overline{Y}_{CkS}$ are the sample means at the Sth analysis given by $\overline{Y}_{TkS} = \sum_{i=1}^{n_S} Y_{Tki}/n_S$ and $\overline{Y}_{CkS} = \sum_{j=1}^{n_S} Y_{Ckj}/n_S$. The same critical boundaries based on any group-sequential methods utilized for the case without sample size recalculation are used.

The sample size is increased or decreased when the conditional power (CP) evaluated at the Sth analysis is lower or higher than the desired power $1 - \beta$. Under the planned MSS and a given observed value of (Z_{1S}, Z_{2S}) based on DF-A discussed in Chap. 2, the CP is given by

$$
CP = \begin{cases}
\Pr\left[\bigcup_{m=S+1}^{L} \{Z_{1m} > c_{1m}^E(\alpha)\} \middle| a_{1S}, a_{2l'}\right] \\
\quad \text{if} \quad Z_{1l} \leq c_{1l}^E(\alpha) \ \text{for all} \ l = 1, \ldots, S, \\
\quad \text{and} \quad Z_{2l'} > c_{2l'}^E(\alpha) \ \text{for some} \ l' = 1, \ldots, S, \\[2mm]
\Pr\left[\bigcup_{m=S+1}^{L} \{Z_{2m} > c_{2m}^E(\alpha)\} \middle| a_{2S}, a_{1l'}\right] \\
\quad \text{if} \quad Z_{2l} \leq c_{2l}^E(\alpha) \ \text{for all} \ l = 1, \ldots, S, \\
\quad \text{and} \quad Z_{1l'} > c_{1l'}^E(\alpha) \ \text{for some} \ l' = 1, \ldots, S, \\[2mm]
\Pr\left[\left\{\bigcup_{m=S+1}^{L} \{Z_{1m} > c_{1m}^E(\alpha)\}\right\} \bigcap \left\{\bigcup_{m=S+1}^{L} \{Z_{2m} > c_{2m}^E(\alpha)\}\right\} \middle| a_{1S}, a_{2S}\right] \\
\quad \text{if} \quad Z_{1l} \leq c_{1l}^E(\alpha) \ \text{and} \ Z_{2l} \leq c_{2l}^E(\alpha) \ \text{for all} \ l = 1, \ldots, S,
\end{cases}
$$

$$(3.1)$$

where (a_{1S}, a_{2S}) is a given observed value of (Z_{1S}, Z_{2S}). On the other hand, if $Z_{1l} \leq c_{1l}^E(\alpha)$ or $Z_{2l} \leq c_{2l}^E(\alpha)$ for all $l = 1, \ldots, S$, then the CP for DF-B is defined by

$$\mathrm{CP} = \Pr\left[\bigcup_{m=S+1}^{L}\left\{\{Z_{1m} > c_{1m}^{\mathrm{E}}(\alpha)\}\bigcap\{Z_{2m} > c_{2m}^{\mathrm{E}}(\alpha)\}\right\}\bigg|a_{1S}, a_{2S}\right], \qquad (3.2)$$

The detailed calculation of the CPs based on DF-A and DF-B is provided in the Appendix B. Since (Δ_1, Δ_2) is unknown, it is customary to substitute (Δ_1^*, Δ_2^*), the estimated mean differences at the Sth analysis $(\widehat{\Delta}_{1S}, \widehat{\Delta}_{2S})$ or the assumed mean differences during trial planning $(\widetilde{\Delta}_1, \widetilde{\Delta}_2)$. We consider the CP based on $(\Delta_1^*, \Delta_2^*) = (\widehat{\Delta}_{1S}, \widehat{\Delta}_{2S})$, which allows the evaluation of behavior of power independent of $(\widetilde{\Delta}_1, \widetilde{\Delta}_2)$.

When recalculating the sample size, three options are possible: (i) only allowing an increase in the sample size, (ii) only allowing a decrease in the sample size, and (iii) allowing an increase or decrease in the sample size. For all of the cases, we assign Z'_{km} and n'_m instead of Z_{km} and n_m in the CPs (3.1) and (3.2). Consider the rule for determining the recalculated sample size n'_L, when the sample size may be increased only, which is:

$$n'_L = \begin{cases} n_L, & \text{if CP} \geq 1 - \beta \text{ or min}(\widehat{\Delta}_{1S}, \widehat{\Delta}_{2S}) \leq 0, \\ \min(n''_L, \lambda n_L), & \text{otherwise.} \end{cases}$$

where n''_L is the smallest integer $n'_L (> n_S)$, where the CP achieves the desired power $1 - \beta$. When the sample size may be decreased only, the recalculated sample size n'_L is given as:

$$n'_L = \begin{cases} n''_L, & \text{if CP} \geq 1 - \beta, \\ n_L, & \text{otherwise.} \end{cases}$$

When the sample size may be increased or decreased, the recalculated sample size n'_L is given as:

$$n'_L = \begin{cases} n''_L, & \text{if CP} > 1 - \beta, \\ n_L, & \text{if CP} = 1 - \beta \text{ or min}(\widehat{\Delta}_{1S}, \widehat{\Delta}_{2S}) \leq 0, \\ \min(n''_L, \lambda n_L), & \text{otherwise.} \end{cases}$$

Incorporating the uncertainty of the estimates at the interim into the sample size recalculation is important in practice. When planning the sample size recalculation in clinical trials with multiple co-primary endpoints, one practical question is whether the sample size is increased or decreased in sample size recalculation. Referring to Asakura et al. (2014), the option of decreasing the sample size is not good choice as the power cannot maintain the targeted power although the expected sample size can be reduced more than the other recalculation options. For other options, i.e., only allowing an increase in the sample size or allowing an increase or decrease in the sample size, the targeted power is maintained.

An important decision regards the optimal timing of the sample size recalculation. The timing should also be carefully considered as the power does not reach desired levels if the sample size recalculation is done too early in the trial, especially when considering a decrease in the sample size. For more details, please see Asakura et al. (2014).

3.3 Illustration

We provide an example to illustrate the sample size recalculation discussed in Sect. 3.2. The tarenflurbil study (Green et al. 2009) is again used to illustrate the sample size recalculation. Recall that the study was designed to evaluate whether tarenflurbil is superior to placebo on cognitive decline and activities of daily living in patients with mild Alzheimer's disease. Co-primary endpoints were cognition as assessed by ADAS-Cog (EP1) and functional ability was as assessed by ADCS–ADL (EP2).

Table 3.1 summarized the recalculated sample size based on the five scenarios of the observed effect $(\widehat{\Delta}_{1S}, \widehat{\Delta}_{2S})$ in a group-sequential clinical trial with two analyses $(L = 2)$, where the decision-making for rejecting H_0 is based on DF-A. The planned MSS is calculated to detect the joint effect on both endpoints assuming the standardized mean difference $(\widetilde{\Delta}_1, \widetilde{\Delta}_2) = (0.20, 0.20)$, correlation $\rho_T = \rho_C = \rho = 0.0$ and 0.80, with 80 % power at 2.5 % significance level for a one-sided test. The critical boundaries are determined by the O'Brien–Fleming-type boundary (OF) (O'Brien and Fleming 1979), using Lan–DeMets error-spending method (Lan and DeMets 1983) with the information time of 0.25, 0.50, and 0.75. The sample size is recalculated based on the three options: (a) only increasing the sample size, (b) only decreasing the sample size, and (c) increasing or decreasing the sample size, with a prespecified constant for the maximum allowable sample size $\lambda = 1.5$. The five scenarios are as follows: (i) both standardized mean differences at the interim are the same as those at the planning, (ii) both standardized mean differences at the interim are larger than those at the planning, (iii) standardized mean differences at the interim are smaller than those at the planning, (iv) only the standardized mean difference for the ADAS-Cog at the interim is larger than that at the planning, and (v) only the standardized mean difference for the ADCS–ADL at the interim is smaller than that at the planning.

In all of the five scenarios and the three options for sample size recalculation, the sample sizes recalculated at the interim of 0.25 information time are larger than those at the interim of 0.50 information time. At the interim corresponding to 0.70 information time, except for scenarios (iii) and (v), sample size recalculation is not performed when the joint statistical significance on both endpoints has been established. At the interim corresponding to 0.25 or 0.50 information time, if the observed standardized mean difference for either of endpoints is larger than assumed, Option (b) or (c) suggests decreasing the sample size, but Option (a) suggests no change in the sample size. However, if the sample size is decreased in such a situation, then the power is always lower than the desired power,

Table 3.1 Recalculated sample size based on the five scenarios of the observed effect $(\widehat{\Delta}_{1S}, \widehat{\Delta}_{2S})$ in a group-sequential clinical trial with two analyses ($L = 2$), where the decision-making is based on DF-A

Timing of recalculation: information time	Scenario: observed effect at the interim $(\widehat{\Delta}_{1S}, \widehat{\Delta}_{2S})$		$\rho = 0.0$				$\rho = 0.8$			
			Planned MSS	(a)	(b)	(c)	Planned MSS	(a)	(b)	(c)
0.25	(i)	(0.20, 0.20)	516	516	464	464	458	458	416	416
	(ii)	(0.25, 0.25)		516	307	307		458	275	275
	(iii)	(0.15, 0.15)		774	516	774		687	458	687
	(iv)	(0.25, 0.20)		516	464	464		458	369	369
	(v)	(0.20, 0.15)		677	516	677		651	458	651
0.50	(i)	(0.20, 0.20)	518	518	414	414	460	460	376	376
	(ii)	(0.25, 0.25)		518	305	305		460	274	274
	(iii)	(0.15, 0.15)		741	518	741		677	458	687
	(iv)	(0.25, 0.20)		518	364	364		460	342	342
	(v)	(0.20, 0.15)		604	518	604		593	460	593
0.75	(i)	(0.20, 0.20)	525	–	–	–	467	–	–	–
	(ii)	(0.25, 0.25)		–	–	–		–	–	–
	(iii)	(0.15, 0.15)		630	525	630		593	467	593
	(iv)	(0.25, 0.20)		–	–	–		–	–	–
	(v)	(0.20, 0.15)		526	525	526		531	467	531

The planned MSS is calculated to detect the joint effect on both endpoints assuming the standardized mean difference $(\widetilde{\Delta}_1, \widetilde{\Delta}_2) = (0.20, 0.20)$, and correlation $\rho_T = \rho_C = \rho = 0.0$ and 0.80, with 80 % power at 2.5 % significance level for a one-sided test. The critical boundaries are determined by the OF, using Lan–DeMets error-spending method with the information time of 0.25, 0.50, and 0.75. The sample size is recalculated based on the three options: (a) only increasing the sample size, (b) only decreasing the sample size, and (c) increasing or decreasing the sample size, with a prespecified constant for the maximum allowable sample size $\lambda = 1.5$. The five scenarios are as follows: (i) both standardized mean differences at the interim are the same as those at the planning, (ii) both standardized mean differences at the interim are larger than those at the planning, (iii) standardized mean differences at the interim are smaller than those at the planning, (iv) only the standardized mean difference for the ADAS-Cog (EP1) at the interim is larger than that at the planning, and (v) only the standardized mean difference for the ADCS–ADL (EP2) at the interim is smaller than that at the planning
–: Sample size recalculation is not performed when the joint statistical significance on both endpoints has been established

especially with higher correlation (Asakura et al. 2014). Based on these results, the timing of the sample size recalculation should be carefully considered as the power does not reach desired levels if the sample size recalculation is carried out early in the trial when considering a decrease in the sample size.

3.4 Application to Binary Outcomes

Consider application of the sample size calculation methods discussed in the previous section for binary outcomes. For illustration, consider the simplest situation, i.e., the two-stage group-sequential design with one interim and final analyses.

The CHW test statistics based on independent samples at the interim and final analyses Z_{k1} and Z''_{k2} are given by

$$Z_{k1} = \frac{\sqrt{n_1}\,\hat{\delta}_{k1}}{\sqrt{2\hat{\bar{p}}_{k1}\,\hat{\bar{q}}_{k1}}} \quad \text{and} \quad Z''_{k2} = \frac{\sqrt{n''_2 - n_1}\,\hat{\delta}''_{k2}}{\sqrt{2\hat{\bar{p}}''_{k2}\,\hat{\bar{q}}''_{k2}}},$$

where $\hat{\delta}''_{k2} = (n'_2 - n_1)^{-1}(\sum_{i=n_1+1}^{n'_2} Y_{Tki} - \sum_{j=n_1+1}^{n'_2} Y_{Ckj})$, $\hat{\bar{q}}_{k1} = 1 - \hat{\bar{p}}_{k1}$, and $\hat{\bar{q}}''_{k2} = 1 - \hat{\bar{p}}''_{k2}$. Therefore, the CHW statistics are $Z'_{k2} = w_1 Z_{k1} + w_2 Z''_{k2}$, where $w_1 = \sqrt{n_1/n_2}$ and $w_2 = \sqrt{(n_2 - n_1)/n_2}$.

Using these test statistics, the sample size is increased or decreased when the CP evaluated at the Sth analysis is lower or higher than the desired power $1 - \beta$. Under the planned MSS and a given observed value of (Z_{1S}, Z_{2S}) based on DF-A and DF-B, the CPs are given by the same forms given in (3.1) and (3.2). For more details, please see Asakura et al. (2015).

The PLACIDE study (Allen et al. 2012, 2013) is again used to illustrate the sample size recalculation. Recall that the study was a double-blind, randomized, parallel-group placebo-controlled trial evaluating lactobacilli and bifidobacteria for the prevention of antibiotic-associated diarrhea in older people admitted to the hospital. The MSS based on DF-A and DF-B is 1146 per intervention group based on an alternative hypothesis of differences for both antibiotic-associated diarrhea (AAD) ($\delta_1 = -0.10$ with $p_{C1} = 0.20$) and C *difficile* diarrhea (CDD) ($\delta_2 = -0.02$ with $p_{C2} = 0.04$), $\rho_T = \rho_C = \rho = 0.0, 0.3, 0.5$ and 0.8, with an alternative hypothesis of differences in proportions to AAD ($p_{T1} = 0.2$ and $p_{C1} = 0.4$) and CDD ($p_{T2} = 0.02$ and $p_{C2} = 0.04$) with 80 % power at 2.5 % significance level for one-sided test, using the normal approximation method, where the critical boundaries are determined by the OF for both endpoints, using the Lan–DeMets error-spending method with equally spaced increments of information.

When considering the same three options based on the rule for determining the recalculated sample size n'_L mentioned in Sect. 3.1, Table 3.2 displays the recalculated sample sizes, CPs and empirical CP (ECP)s based on DF-A and DF-B under the five scenarios, i.e., (i) both differences in proportions at the interim are same as those at the planning, (ii) both differences in proportions at the interim are smaller than those at the planning, (iii) both differences in proportions at the interim are larger than those at the planning, (iv) only the difference in proportions for the AAD at the interim is smaller than that at the planning, and (v) only the difference in proportions for the CDD at the interim is smaller than that at the planning. The ECP is evaluated via Monte Carlo simulation with the 100,000 runs for each scenario. The bivariate Bernoulli data for the Monte Carlo simulation were generated by the method in Emrich and Piedmonte (1991). The sample size is recalculated when the CP evaluated at the interim analysis is lower or higher than the desired power $1 - \beta$ under the three options: (a) only increasing the sample size, (b) only decreasing the sample size, and (c) increasing or decreasing the sample size, with a prespecified constant for the maximum allowable sample size $\lambda = 1.5$ and $\rho_T = \rho_C = \rho = 0.0$,

Table 3.2 The recalculated sample sizes, CP and ECP under the five scenarios, where the decision-making is based on DF-A and the scenarios are (i) both differences in proportions at the interim are the same as those at the planning, (ii) both differences in proportions at the interim are smaller than those at the planning, (iii) both differences in proportions at the interim are larger than those at the planning, (iv) only the difference in proportions for the AAD at the interim is smaller than that at the planning, and (v) only the difference in proportions for the CDD at the interim is smaller than that at the planning

Scenario: observed effect at the interim $(\hat{\delta}_{1S}, \hat{\delta}_{2S})$		Option	Before recalculation		After recalculation		
			CP(%)	ECP(%)	n'_L	CP(%)	ECP(%)
(i)	(0.10, 0.02)	(a)	88.2	88.8	1146	88.2	88.8
		(b)	88.2	88.8	968	80.2	80.8
		(c)	88.2	88.8	968	80.2	80.8
(ii)	(0.05, 0.01)	(a)	54.8	55.2	1719	82.8	83.3
		(b)	54.8	55.2	1146	54.8	55.2
		(c)	54.8	55.2	1719	82.8	83.3
(iii)	(0.15, 0.025)	(a)	96.3	96.2	1146	96.3	96.2
		(b)	96.3	96.2	669	73.1	72.7
		(c)	96.3	96.2	669	73.1	72.7
(iv)	(0.05, 0.02)	(a)	88.2	88.8	1146	88.2	88.8
		(b)	88.2	88.8	1074	85.5	85.9
		(c)	88.2	88.8	1074	85.5	85.9
(v)	(0.10 0.01)	(a)	54.8	55.3	1719	82.8	83.6
		(b)	54.8	55.3	1146	54.8	55.3
		(c)	54.8	55.3	1719	82.8	83.6

The sample size is recalculated when the CP evaluated at the interim analysis is lower or higher than the desired power $1 - \beta$ under the three options: (a) only increasing the sample size, (b) only decreasing the sample size, and (c) increasing or decreasing the sample size, with a prespecified constant for the maximum allowable sample size $\lambda = 1.5$ and $\rho_T = \rho_C = \rho = 0.0$, where the critical boundaries for both endpoints are determined by the OF, using the Lan–DeMets error-spending method with equally spaced increments of information

where the critical boundaries for both endpoints are determined by the OF, using the Lan–DeMets error-spending method with equally spaced increments of information.

In all scenarios of observed interim effects, when only allowing an increase in the sample size, the CP (and ECP) is always higher than 80 % desired power. When allowing an increase or a decrease in the sample size, except for scenario (iii) of both differences in proportions at the interim are larger than those at the planning, the CPs are always larger than 80 % power. On the other hand, when only allowing a decrease in the sample size, the CPs are always lower than the desired power. In this example, the sample size recalculation is supposed to be conducted at the information time of 0.50. As discussed in the previous sections, the timing of sample size recalculation is important. The power is much lower than desired power if the sample size recalculation is conducted early in the trial, especially when allowing for a decrease in the sample size.

3.5 Summary

As with group-sequential trials involving a single primary endpoint, designing group-sequential trials with co-primary endpoints can provide efficiencies by detecting trends prior to planned completion of the trial. It may also be prudent to evaluate design assumptions at the interim and potentially make design adjustments (i.e., sample size recalculation) if design assumptions were dramatically inaccurate. In this chapter, we discuss sample size recalculation based on the observed intervention's effects at an interim analysis with a focus on control of statistical error rates.

References

Allen SJ, Wareham K, Bradley C, Harris W, Dhar A, Brown H, Foden A, Cheung WY, Gravenor MB, Plummer S, Phillips CJ, Mack D (2012) A multicentre randomised controlled trial evaluating lactobacilli and bifidobacteria in the prevention of antibiotic-associated diarrhoea in older people admitted to hospital: the PLACIDE study protocol. BMC Infect Dis 12:108

Allen SJ, Wareham K, Wang D, Bradley C, Hutchings H, Harris W, Dhar A, Brown H, Foden A, Gravenor MB, Mack D (2013) Lactobacilli and bifidobacteria in the prevention of antibiotic-associated diarrhoea and Clostridium difficile diarrhoea in older inpatients (PLACIDE): a randomised, double-blind, placebo-controlled, multicentre trial. Lancet 382:1249–1257

Asakura K, Hamasaki T, Sugimoto T, Hayashi K, Evans SR, Sozu T (2014) Sample size determination in group-sequential clinical trials with two co-primary endpoints. Stat Med 33:2897–2913

Asakura K, Hamasaki T, Evans SR, Sugimoto T, Sozu T (2015) Sample size determination in group-sequential clinical trials with two co-primary endpoints. In: Chen Z, Liu A, Qu Y, Tang L, Ting N, Tsong Y (eds) Applied statistics in bio-medicine and clinical trial design (Chap. 14). Springer International Publishing, Cham, pp 235–262

Cui L, Hung HMJ, Wang SJ (1999) Modification of sample size in group sequential clinical trials. Biometrics 55:853–857

Emrich LJ, Piedmonte MR (1991) A method for generating high-dimensional multivariate binary variates. Am Stat 45:302–304

Green R, Schneider LS, Amato DA, Beelen AP, Wilcock G, Swabb EA, Zavitz KH, for the Tarenflurbil Phase 3 Study Group (2009) Effect of tarenflurbil on cognitive decline and activities of daily living in patients with mild Alzheimer disease: a randomized controlled trial. J Am Med Assoc 302:2557–2564

Lan KKG, DeMets DL (1983) Discrete sequential boundaries for clinical trials. Biometrika 70:659–663

O'Brien PC, Fleming TR (1979) A multiple testing procedure for clinical trials. Biometrics 35:549–556

Chapter 4
Interim Evaluation of Efficacy or Futility in Clinical Trials with Two Co-primary Endpoints

Abstract We discuss group-sequential designs for early efficacy or futility stopping in superiority clinical trials with multiple co-primary endpoints. We discuss several decision-making frameworks for evaluating efficacy or futility based on boundaries using group-sequential methodology. We incorporate the correlations among the endpoints into the calculations for futility critical boundaries and evaluate the required sample sizes as a function of design parameters including mean differences, the number of planned analyses, and efficacy critical boundaries. We provide an example to illustrate the methods and discuss practical considerations when designing efficient group-sequential designs in clinical trials with co-primary endpoints.

Keywords Error-spending method · Futility · Multiple endpoints · Non-binding boundary · Type I error · Type II error

4.1 Introduction

In this chapter, we consider group-sequential designs in clinical trials with multiple co-primary endpoints with the decision-making frameworks for rejecting the null or alternative hypothesis (i.e., early stopping for either efficacy or futility).

In addition to early stopping for efficacy assessment as discussed in Chap. 2, it can be equally important to monitor the clinical trials to assess the futility, e.g., when an intervention that is being investigated is not working. The tarenflurbil trial (Green et al. 2009) mentioned in Chap. 2 unfortunately failed to demonstrate a beneficial effect of tarenflurbil on both the Alzheimer's Disease Assessment Scale Cognitive Subscale (ADAS-Cog) and the Alzheimer's Disease Cooperative Study Activities of Daily Living (ADCS-ADL). The observed treatment effect estimates were smaller than the assumed effects. In fact, the observed ADCS-ADL in the tarenflurbil group was smaller than that for the placebo group. If the design had included a futility assessment, the clinical trial may have been stopped based on an interim result suggesting that the treatment was not effective and it was unlikely to demonstrate a desirable result. This may have saved resources and time, and

© The Author(s) 2016
51
T. Hamasaki et al., *Group-Sequential Clinical Trials with Multiple Co-Objectives*,
JSS Research Series in Statistics, DOI 10.1007/978-4-431-55900-9_4

prevented patients from being exposed to an ineffective intervention unnecessarily (Gould and Pecore 1982; Ware et al. 1985; Snapinn et al. 2006).

There are two fundamental approaches for assessing futility: based on the conditional probability of rejecting the null hypothesis (Lan et al. 1982; Lachin 2005) and based on the critical boundaries using group-sequential methodology (DeMets and Ware 1980, 1982; Chang et al. 1998; Whitehead and Matsushita 2003). In this chapter, we focus on the latter as we have discussed conditional probability in Chap. 3 and develop the method as an extension of Jennison and Turnbull (1993), and Cook and Farewell (1994), where they discussed the decision-making frameworks associated with interim evaluation of efficacy and futility to monitor the efficacy and safety responses, and considered a simple method for determining the boundaries. The approach must preserve the desired Type I and Type II error rates, α and β analogously to the single endpoint case. When planning interim efficacy assessments in clinical trials with multiple co-primary endpoints, the efficacy boundary is usually determined separately using group-sequential methods [e.g., Lan–DeMets error-spending method (Lan and DeMets 1983)] to control the Type I error, analogous to the single primary endpoint case (Asakura et al. 2014). However, the efficacy boundary could be adjusted by incorporating the correlations among the endpoints [Chuang-Stein et al. (2007) and Kordzakhia et al. (2010) discussed this for fixed-sample designs]. This strategy may provide smaller sample sizes but also introduces challenges. The sample size calculated to detect the joint effect may be smaller than the sample size calculated for each individual endpoint. Furthermore, the correlation is usually unknown and estimates from prior studies may be incorrect. This calls into question whether or not the significance level should be adjusted based on the unknown nuisance parameter. On the other hand, when planning for interim futility assessment in trials with multiple co-primary endpoints, it is unclear how adjusting the futility boundary by incorporating the correlations may affect the decision-making for accepting the null hypothesis although Jennison and Turnbull (1993) provide the fundamentals on this issue. We investigate this issue by evaluating the operating characteristics in terms of efficacy and futility boundaries, power, the Type I error, and sample sizes, as a function of mean differences, correlation, and the number of analyses.

Using the notation defined in Chap. 2, we consider a two-arm parallel group trial designed to evaluate whether a test intervention (T) is superior to a control (C) based on two continuous outcomes EP1 and EP2 ($K = 2$) as co-primary endpoints. Suppose that a maximum of L analyses are planned, where the same number of planned analyses with the same information space is selected for both endpoints. Let n_l and $r_C n_l$ be the cumulative number of participants on the T and the C at the lth analysis ($l = 1, \ldots, L$), respectively, where r_C is the allocation ratio of the C to the T. Hence, up to n_L and $r_C n_L$, participants are recruited and randomly assigned to the T and the C, respectively. Then, there are n_L paired outcomes (Y_{T1i}, Y_{T2i}) ($i = 1, \ldots, n_L$) for the T and $r_C n_L$ paired outcomes (Y_{C1j}, Y_{C2j}) ($j = 1, \ldots, r_C n_L$) for the C.

Assume that (Y_{T1i}, Y_{T2i}) and (Y_{C1j}, Y_{C2j}) are independently bivariate-distributed with means $E[Y_{Tki}] = \mu_{Tk}$ and $E[Y_{Ckj}] = \mu_{Ck}$, variances $\text{var}[Y_{Tki}] = \sigma_{Tk}^2$ and $\text{var}[Y_{Ckj}] = \sigma_{Ck}^2$, and correlations $\text{corr}[Y_{T1i}, Y_{T2i}] = \rho_T$ and $\text{corr}[Y_{C1j}, Y_{C2j}] = \rho_C$, respectively $(k = 1, 2)$. For simplicity, the variances are assumed to be known and common, i.e., $\sigma_{Tk}^2 = \sigma_{Ck}^2 = \sigma_k^2$. There is an interest in testing $H_0: H_{01} \cup H_{02}$ versus $H_1: H_{11} \cap H_{12}$ at the α level within the context of group-sequential designs, where $H_{0k}: \delta_k \leq 0$ and $H_{1k}: \delta_k > 0$ with $\delta_k = \mu_{Tk} - \mu_{Ck}$.

4.2 Decision-Making Frameworks and Stopping Rules

We describe the decision-making frameworks with associated rules for rejecting or accepting the H_0 when implementing both efficacy and futility assessments.

When assessing futility on two co-primary endpoints in a group-sequential setting, the decision-making rule is to accept H_0 if the test statistic for *at least one* endpoint crosses a prespecified group-sequential-based futility critical boundary at any interim analysis. If the trial is not stopped when at least one test statistic has crossed the futility critical boundary, then the Type I error will be inflated analogously to trials with a single primary endpoint. We only discuss the non-binding futility critical boundary, assuming that the trial is stopped when at least one test statistic has crossed the futility critical boundary, although the binding futility critical boundary may be used in this situation.

When assessing efficacy, as discussed in Chap. 2, there are two options for testing H_0 (Asakura et al. 2014, 2015; Chen et al. 2014; Hamasaki et al. 2015; Ando et al. 2015). One is to reject H_0 if each test statistic crosses the prespecified group-sequential-based efficacy critical boundary at any interim analysis (i.e., not necessarily simultaneously), but both the test statistics should cross the critical boundary at each analysis until completion of the trial. If either of the test statistics crosses the critical boundary at an interim analysis, then the trial continues, but subsequent hypothesis testing is repeatedly conducted only for the previously non-significant endpoint. The other option is a special case of the first one: reject H_0 if both the test statistics cross the critical boundary at an interim analysis simultaneously. If either of the test statistics does not cross the critical boundary, then the trial continues until all of the test statistics cross the critical boundary simultaneously.

By combining the two decision-making rules for efficacy assessment with the decision-making rule for futility assessment, we consider an option that allows selecting different numbers and timings for interim analyses for efficacy and futility assessments. For example, three analyses for efficacy assessment (with information times of 0.50, 0.75, and 1.0) and two analyses for futility assessment (with information times of 0.25 and 1.0) could be conducted. This provides an opportunity for detecting an early negative sign for either of the endpoints, but also has flexibility for delaying efficacy analyses to improve the power.

For example, based on our recent observations in developing drugs for the treatment of Alzheimer's disease, it seems more difficult to detect the effect on functional or global endpoint [e.g., Alzheimer's Disease Cooperative Study Clinician's Global Impression of Change (ADCS-CGIS), Clinician's Interview-Based Impression of Change, plus caregiver (CIBIC-plus)], rather than cognitive endpoint (ADAS-cog). Functional or global endpoint generally requires a larger sample size as the effect is smaller than the cognitive endpoint. In fact, the three phase III confirmatory clinical trials of rivastigmine, memantine, and galantamine, which were conducted in Japan, failed to demonstrate a significant beneficial effect on functional or global endpoint (Pharmaceuticals and Medical Devices Agency, PMDA 2010a, b, 2011) although the effects on functional or global endpoint were positive compared with placebo. One possible strategy for evaluating the effect of drugs for the treatment of Alzheimer's disease is to assess futility only for the cognitive endpoint at an early interim analysis and to assess the efficacy for both cognitive and functional or global endpoints at late interim analyses if negative signs are not detected for the cognitive endpoint during the earlier interim analyses. If a negative sign is detected for the cognitive endpoint at the earlier interim analysis, then the clinical trial is terminated.

Based on these concepts, we describe three decision-making frameworks with corresponding stopping rules and power definitions.

DF-A: The first decision-making framework, DF-A, is to (i) accept H_0 if the test statistic for at least one endpoint crosses a prespecified group-sequential-based futility critical boundary at any interim analysis and (ii) to reject H_0 if each test statistic crosses the prespecified group-sequential-based efficacy critical boundary at any interim analysis (i.e., not necessarily simultaneously). Here, suppose that L_k analyses are planned for efficacy or futility assessments for endpoint k, and the total number of planned analyses L is the sum of the number of planned analyses over all endpoints, excluding the duplications of the same information time $n_{l_k}/n_L(=I_{l_k}) = n_{l_{k'}}/n_L(=I_{l_{k'}})$ $(l_k = 1,\ldots,L_k;\ l_{k'} = 1,\ldots,L_{k'};\ 1 \leq L_{k'},\ L_k \leq L)$. The stopping rule based on DF-A is formally given as follows:

Until the lth analysis $(l = 1,\ldots,L-1)$,

if $Z_{kl_k} \leq c_{kl_k}^{F}(\beta)$ for at least one endpoint, for some $1 \leq l_k \leq l$, then accept H_0 and stop the trial,
if $Z_{kl_k} > c_{kl_k}^{E}(\alpha)$ for both endpoints, for some $1 \leq l_k \leq l$, then reject H_0 and stop the trial,
otherwise, continue to the $(l+1)$th analysis,

at the Lth analysis,

if $Z_{kL_k} \leq c_{kL_k}^{F}(\beta)$ for at least one endpoint, then do not reject H_0,
if $Z_{kL_k} > c_{kL_k}^{E}(\alpha)$ for the non-significant endpoint(s) until the $(L-1)$th analysis, then reject H_0,

where Z_{kl_k} is the test statistic for kth endpoint at the l_kth analysis

$$Z_{kl_k} = \frac{\overline{Y}_{Tkl_k} - \overline{Y}_{Ckl_k}}{\sigma_k \sqrt{(1 + 1/r_C)/n_{l_k}}},$$

where $\overline{Y}_{Tkl_k}$ and $\overline{Y}_{Ckl_k}$ are the sample means for T and C for the l_kth analysis defined in Chap. 2. Also, $c_{kl_k}^E(\alpha)$ and $c_{kl_k}^F(\beta)$ are the efficacy and futility critical boundaries, determined using any group-sequential method, respectively. The power for detecting the joint effect on both endpoints, corresponding to the DF-A, is

$$1 - \beta = \Pr\left[\bigcap_{k=1}^{2}\left\{A_{k1} \cup \bigcup_{l_k=2}^{L_k}\left\{\bigcap_{l_k'=1}^{l_k-1} B_{kl_k'} \cap A_{kl_k}\right\}\right\}\Big|H_1\right]. \tag{4.1}$$

where $A_{kl_k} = \left\{Z_{kl_k} > c_{kl_k}^E(\alpha)\right\}$ and $B_{kl_k} = \left\{c_{kl_k}^F(\beta) < Z_{kl_k} \leq c_{kl_k}^E(\alpha)\right\}$.

As mentioned in Chap. 2, the efficacy critical boundaries $c_{kl_k}^E(\alpha)$ are constant and determined separately, using any group-sequential method to control the Type I error rate, analogous to the single primary endpoint case. The futility critical boundaries $c_{kl_k}^F(\beta)$ are also constant and determined for achieving the desired power $1 - \beta$ and controlling the marginal Type I error rate to the prespecified level α with $c_{kL}^F(\beta) = c_{kL}^E(\alpha)$ at the final analysis, using any group-sequential method. The efficacy and futility boundaries at the first analysis $c_{k1}^E(\alpha)$ and $c_{k1}^F(\beta)$ are determined such that:

$$\Pr\left[Z_{k1} > c_{k1}^E(\alpha)|H_0\right] = f_k(\mathcal{J}_1) \text{ and } \Pr\left[Z_{k1} \leq c_{k1}^F(\alpha)|H_1\right] = g_k(\mathcal{J}_1),$$

where $f_k(\mathcal{J}_l)$ and $g_k(\mathcal{J}_l)$ are error-spending functions for endpoint k, which describes the error rates spent until the lth analysis with the information time $\mathcal{J}_l$ and $f_k(0) = g_k(0) = 0$ and $f_k(1) = \alpha$ and $g_k(1) = \beta_k$. At the subsequent analyses, $c_{kl}^E(\alpha)$ and $c_{kl}^F(\beta)$ are determined satisfying

$$\Pr\left[Z_{k1} \leq c_{k1}^E(\alpha), \ldots, Z_{kl-1} \leq c_{kl-1}^E(\alpha),\, Z_{kl} > c_{kl}^E(\alpha)|H_0\right] = f_k(\mathcal{J}_l) - f_k(\mathcal{J}_{l-1})$$

and

$$\Pr\left[c_{k1}^F(\beta) < Z_{k1} \leq c_{k1}^E(\alpha), \ldots, c_{kl-1}^F(\beta) < Z_{kl-1} \leq c_{kl-1}^E(\alpha),\, Z_{kl} \leq c_{kl}^F(\beta)|H_1\right]$$
$$= g_k(\mathcal{J}_l) - g_k(\mathcal{J}_{l-1}).$$

For the method for calculating the efficacy and futility boundaries, see Asakura et al. (2015).

Figure 4.1 displays the efficacy and futility critical boundaries for the DF-A in a group-sequential clinical trial with the four planned analyses ($L = 4$). The efficacy and futility assessments are conducted for the two endpoints at the same interim analysis. Both efficacy and futility critical boundaries are determined by the O'Brien–Fleming-type boundary (OF) (O'Brien and Fleming 1979), using Lan–DeMets error-spending method, for spending the Type I and II errors, with equally spaced increments of information, where the trial is designed to detect a joint effect on both endpoints [the standardized mean differences $(\Delta_1, \Delta_2) = (0.1, 0.1)$, $(0.1, 0.2)$ and $(0.2, 0.2)$] with 80 % power at 2.5 % significance level for a one-sided test, where $\Delta_k = \delta_k / \sigma_k (k = 1, 2)$.

The figure illustrates that the regions based on the efficacy and futility critical boundaries for the two endpoints are narrower when the standardized mean differences are larger and when the correlation is larger. When $\Delta_1 = \Delta_2$, the futility critical boundaries for both endpoints vary with the correlation.

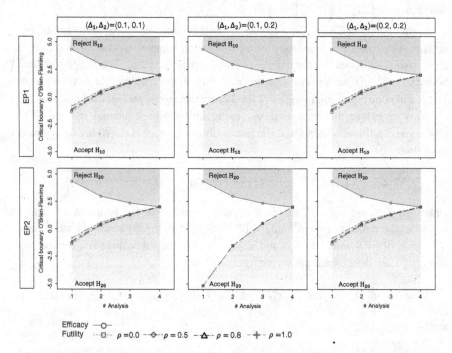

Fig. 4.1 Efficacy and futility critical boundaries with correlation and standardized mean differences in a group-sequential clinical trial with two analyses ($L = 4$), where the decision-making is based on DF-A. The trial is designed to detect a joint effect on both endpoints with 80 % power at a 2.5 % significance level for a one-sided test. The standardized mean differences are $(\Delta_1, \Delta_2) = (0.1, 0.1), (0.1, 0.2)$ and $(0.2, 0.2)$. The efficacy and futility assessments are conducted for the two endpoints at the same interim analyses. The critical boundaries are determined by the OF, using the Lan–DeMets error-spending method with equally spaced increments of information

If $\rho_T = \rho_C = \rho = 0.0$, then the futility critical boundaries for both endpoints are equal to the ones individually calculated for each endpoint with the power of $\sqrt{1-\beta} = 89.4\%$ and ones with 80 % power if $\rho = 1.0$. When $\Delta_1 < \Delta_2$, the futility critical boundaries do not vary with the correlation. For example, when $(\Delta_1, \Delta_2) = (0.1, 0.2)$, the futility critical boundaries for EP1 are -0.822, 0.609, 1.401, and 2.014 for each analysis and are equal to those calculated for EP1 to detect $\Delta_1 = 0.1$ with 80 % power. On the other hand, for EP2, the futility critical boundaries are $-5.140, -1.504, 0.542$ and 2.014 for each analysis. In this situation, the calculated sample size per intervention group is 1782 which is equal to the one calculated for EP1 with $\Delta_1 = 0.1$ and 80 % power. The futility critical boundaries for EP2 are equal to those calculated to detect Δ_2 with the marginal power for EP2 under this sample size. The method for calculating the efficacy and futility critical boundaries is discussed in the Appendix A3.

DF-B: The second framework, DF-B, is a special case of the DF-A. A major difference in the decision-making rule is to reject H_0 if both of the test statistics cross the critical boundary at the same interim analysis simultaneously. The stopping rule is formally given as follows:

At the lth analysis $(l = 1, \ldots, L-1)$,

if $Z_{kl_k} \leq c^F_{kl_k}(\beta)$ for at least one endpoint, then accept H_0 and stop the trial,
if $Z_{kl_k} > c^E_{kl_k}(\alpha)$ for all endpoints, then reject H_0 and stop the trial,
otherwise, continue to the $(l+1)$th analysis,

at the Lth analysis,

if $Z_{kL_k} \leq c^F_{kL_k}(\beta)$ for at least one endpoint, then do not reject H_0,
if $Z_{kL_k} > c^E_{kL_k}(\alpha)$ for all endpoints, then reject H_0.

Therefore, the power for detecting the joint effect on both endpoints, corresponding to the DF-B, is

$$1 - \beta = \Pr\left[\bigcap_{k=1}^{2} A_{k1} \cup \bigcup_{l_1,\ldots,l_K=2}^{L_1,\ldots,L_K} \left\{\bigcap_{k=1}^{2}\left\{\bigcap_{l'_k=1}^{l_k-1} C_{kl'_k} \cap A_{kl_k}\right\}\right\} \middle| H_1\right], \quad (4.2)$$

where $C_{kl_k} = \left\{Z_{kl_k} > c^F_{kl_k}(\beta)\right\}$.

DF-C: DF-A and DF-B are flexible, but different timings for the interim analyses between the efficacy and futility assessments may introduce operational challenges.

To avoid these difficulties, one may opt for restricting when H_0 is rejected or accepted. The efficacy and futility assessments are simultaneously performed at the same interim analysis, and if the test statistic for at least one endpoint does not cross the prespecified futility critical boundary or if the test statistic for at least one endpoint does not cross the prespecified efficacy critical boundary, then the trial continues until joint significance for all endpoints is established simultaneously. The decision-making framework is same as discussed in Jennison and Turnbull (1993). The stopping rule for the most simplified decision-making framework is formally given as follows:

At the lth analysis $(l = 1, \ldots, L-1)$,

if $Z_{kl} \le c_{kl}^{\mathrm{F}}(\beta)$ for at least one endpoint, accept H_0 and stop the trial,
if $Z_{kl} > c_{kl}^{\mathrm{E}}(\alpha)$ for both endpoints, then reject H_0 and stop the trial,
otherwise, continue to the $(l+1)$th analysis,

at the Lth analysis,

if $Z_{kL} \le c_{kL}^{\mathrm{F}}(\beta)$ for at least one endpoint, do not reject H_0,
if $Z_{kL} > c_{kL}^{\mathrm{E}}(\alpha)$ for both endpoints, then reject H_0.

The corresponding power is

$$1 - \beta = \Pr\left[\bigcap_{k=1}^{2} A_{k1} \cup \bigcup_{l=2}^{L}\left\{\bigcap_{l'=1}^{l-1}\{C_{1l'} \cap C_{2l'}\} \cap \{A_{1l} \cap A_{2l}\}\right\}\Big|H_1\right], \qquad (4.3)$$

where $C_{kl} = \{Z_{kl} > c_{kl}^{\mathrm{F}}(\beta)\}$ and $1 \le l' \le l \le L$.

Asakura et al. (2015) investigate the operating characteristics of these decision-making frameworks in terms of the power, overall Type I error rate, and sample size. In general, DF-A is more powerful than DF-B and DF-C under H_1 (i.e., DF-A requires a smaller sample size than DF-B or DF-C to establish a joint effect on all of the endpoints). In all of the decision-making frameworks, higher correlation increases the power if the standardized mean differences are equal, but does not otherwise affect power. A larger number of planned analyses decrease the power. Allocation of the efficacy and/or futility assessment to an interim analysis with earlier information time increases the power. Higher correlation increases the Type I error rate but not above the targeted significance level. A larger number of futility assessments decrease the Type I error rate. Allocation of the futility assessments to interim analyses with later information time decreases the Type I error rate. For more details, see Asakura et al. (2015).

4.3   Illustration

We illustrate the concepts with an example from the tarenflurbil study (Green et al. 2009) described in Chap. 2. Recall that the study was designed to evaluate whether Tarenflurbil was superior to placebo on two co-primary endpoints, (i) change score from baseline on the ADAS-cog (EP1), and (ii) change score on the ADCS-ADL (EP2). The original design called for 800 participants per intervention group to provide an overall power of 96 % to detect the joint between-group difference in the two primary endpoints using a one-sided test at 2.5 % significance level, with an alternative hypothesis of a standardized mean difference of 0.2 for both endpoints. The correlation between the two endpoints was assumed to be zero.

We discuss the nine group-sequential designs shown in Table 4.1. Five designs include futility and efficacy assessments for both endpoints simultaneously (simultaneous assessment). The last four include a futility assessment for either of the two endpoints (i.e., EP1) only at the first interim analysis and then only efficacy assessments for both endpoints at later interim analyses (separate assessment), where the maximum number of planned analyses is 2, 3, or 4. Tables 4.2, 4.3 and 4.4 display the efficacy and futility critical boundaries, maximum sample size (MSS), and average sample number (ASN) per intervention group (equally sized groups $r_C = 1$) in the DF-A for the group-sequential designs shown in Table 4.1 (For the definition of the MSS and ASN, see Chap. 2.) The MSS was calculated

Table 4.1 Group-sequential designs for efficacy or futility assessment in the tarenflurbil study with two co-primary endpoints, the ADAS-cog (EP1) and the ADCS-ADL (EP2)

Situation	Design #	Assessment	Information time			
			1/4	1/2	3/4	1
1. Simultaneous assessment: efficacy and futility assessments for both endpoints at the same interim analysis simultaneously	#1-1	Efficacy	Both	Both	Both	Both
		Futility	Both	Both	Both	Both
	#1-2	Efficacy		Both	Both	Both
		Futility		Both	Both	Both
	#1-3	Efficacy	Both		Both	Both
		Futility	Both		Both	Both
	#1-4	Efficacy	Both	Both		Both
		Futility	Both	Both		Both
	#1-5	Efficacy		Both		Both
		Futility		Both		Both
2. Separate assessment: futility assessment for EP1 at the first interim analysis and then efficacy assessment for both endpoints at later interim analyses	#2-1	Efficacy		Both	Both	Both
		Futility	EP1			Both
	#2-2	Efficacy			Both	Both
		Futility		EP1		Both
	#2-3	Efficacy			Both	Both
		Futility	EP1			Both
	#2-4	Efficacy		Both		Both
		Futility	EP1			Both

Table 4.2 Efficacy and futility critical boundaries for the group-sequential designs shown in Table 4.1

Design #	Assessment	Correlation ρ	Information time			
			1/4	1/2	3/4	1
#1-1	Efficacy	–	4.333	2.963	2.359	2.014
	Futility	0.0	−2.459	−0.195	1.083	2.014
		0.3	−2.441	−0.186	1.086	2.014
		0.5	−2.412	−0.172	1.092	2.014
		0.8	−2.322	−0.128	1.110	2.014
		1.0	−2.044	0.009	1.165	2.014
#1-2	Efficacy	–	→	2.963	2.359	2.014
	Futility	0.0	→	−0.194	1.083	2.014
		0.3	→	−0.186	1.086	2.014
		0.5	→	−0.172	1.092	2.014
		0.8	→	−0.127	1.110	2.014
		1.0	→	0.010	1.165	2.014
#1-3	Efficacy	–	4.333	→	2.340	2.012
	Futility	0.0	−2.460	→	1.096	2.012
		0.3	−2.442	→	1.100	2.012
		0.5	−2.413	→	1.106	2.012
		0.8	−2.323	→	1.126	2.012
		1.0	−2.048	→	1.187	2.012
#1-4	Efficacy	–	4.333	2.963	→	1.969
	Futility	0.0	−2.492	−0.242	→	1.969
		0.3	−2.471	−0.232	→	1.969
		0.5	−2.446	−0.220	→	1.969
		0.8	−2.355	−0.176	→	1.969
		1.0	−2.080	−0.044	→	1.969
#1-5	Efficacy	–	→	2.963	→	1.969
	Futility	0.0	→	−0.241	→	1.969
		0.3	→	−0.231	→	1.969
		0.5	→	−0.219	→	1.969
		0.8	→	−0.175	→	1.969
		1.0	→	−0.043		1.969

The efficacy and futility assessments are conducted for both endpoints at the same interim analysis simultaneously, where the decision-making is based on DF-A ($\beta = 4\%$ and $\alpha = 2.5\%$)

with an alternative hypothesis of a standardized mean difference for both ADAS-Cog and ADCS-ADL ($\Delta_1 = \Delta_2 = 0.2$), with 96 % power at 2.5 % significance level for a one-sided test, where $\rho_T = \rho_C = \rho = 0.0, 0.3, 0.5, 0.8$ and 1.0. The ASN is calculated under $(\Delta_1, \Delta_2) = (0.2, 0.2), (0.0, 0.2)$ and $(0.0, 0.0)$. The efficacy and futility critical boundaries are determined commonly by the OF, using the Lan–DeMets error-spending method for the Type I and Type II errors with equally or unequally spaced increments of information.

Table 4.3 Efficacy and futility critical boundaries for the group-sequential designs shown in Table 4.1, where the decision-making is based on DF-A

Design #	Assessment	Correlation ρ	Information time			
			1/4	1/2	3/4	1
#2-1	Efficacy	–	$\rightarrow$	2.963	2.359	2.014
	Futility	0.0	−2.482	$\rightarrow$	$\rightarrow$	2.014
		0.3	−2.462	$\rightarrow$	$\rightarrow$	2.014
		0.5	−2.435	$\rightarrow$	$\rightarrow$	2.014
		0.8	−2.343	$\rightarrow$	$\rightarrow$	2.014
		1.0	−2.076	$\rightarrow$	$\rightarrow$	2.014
#2-2	Efficacy	–	$\rightarrow$	$\rightarrow$	2.340	2.012
	Futility	0.0	$\rightarrow$	−0.224	$\rightarrow$	2.012
		0.3	$\rightarrow$	−0.214	$\rightarrow$	2.012
		0.5	$\rightarrow$	−0.201	$\rightarrow$	2.012
		0.8	$\rightarrow$	−0.158	$\rightarrow$	2.012
		1.0	$\rightarrow$	−0.027	$\rightarrow$	2.012
#2-3	Efficacy	–	$\rightarrow$	$\rightarrow$	2.340	2.012
	Futility	0.0	−2.483	$\rightarrow$	$\rightarrow$	2.012
		0.3	−2.463	$\rightarrow$	$\rightarrow$	2.012
		0.5	−2.436	$\rightarrow$	$\rightarrow$	2.012
		0.8	−2.347	$\rightarrow$	$\rightarrow$	2.012
		1.0	−2.076	$\rightarrow$	$\rightarrow$	2.012
#2-4	Efficacy	–	$\rightarrow$	2.963	$\rightarrow$	1.969
	Futility	0.0	−2.495	$\rightarrow$	$\rightarrow$	1.969
		0.3	−2.478	$\rightarrow$	$\rightarrow$	1.969
		0.5	−2.450	$\rightarrow$	$\rightarrow$	1.969
		0.8	−2.357	$\rightarrow$	$\rightarrow$	1.969
		1.0	−2.087	$\rightarrow$	$\rightarrow$	1.969

The futility assessment is conducted for EP1 at the first interim analysis, and then efficacy assessments are conducted for both endpoints at later interim analyses ($\beta = 4\%$ and $\alpha = 2.5\%$). The efficacy and futility critical boundaries are determined commonly by the OF, using the Lan–DeMets error-spending method for the Type I and Type II errors with equally or unequally spaced increments of information

Tables 4.2 and 4.3 illustrate that the regions based on the efficacy and futility critical boundaries for the two endpoints are narrower when the correlation is higher. If the correlation is zero, then the futility critical boundaries for both endpoints are equal to the ones individually calculated for each endpoint with the power of $\sqrt{1 - \beta} = 89.4\%$ and ones with 80 % power if the correlation is one.

When both futility and efficacy assessments are conducted at the same analysis for both endpoints, Table 4.4 shows that the smallest MSS is given by Designs #1-4 or #1-5, but the largest ASN reductions under all of the standardized mean difference combinations are provided by Designs #1-1 or #1-2. When only a futility assessment is conducted at the first interim analysis and then only efficacy

Table 4.4 MSS and ASN (per intervention group) in the group-sequential clinical trials with two co-primary endpoints, including futility and efficacy assessments for the two endpoints for the group-sequential designs shown in Table 4.1, where the decision-making is based on DF-A

Situation	Design #	Correlation ρ	MSS	ASN (Δ_1, Δ_2)		
				(0.2, 0.2)	(0.2, 0.0)	(0.0, 0.0)
1. Simultaneous assessment	#1-1	0.0	836	623	564	489
		0.3	831	608	559	498
		0.5	824	594	553	502
		0.8	798	563	532	500
		1.0	725	498	468	468
	#1-2	0.0	836	623	565	492
		0.3	831	608	561	501
		0.5	824	595	555	505
		0.8	798	564	533	503
		1.0	725	500	472	472
	#1-3	0.0	835	669	650	624
		0.3	829	661	645	623
		0.5	822	654	639	620
		0.8	796	629	617	606
		1.0	722	566	554	554
	#1-4	0.0	809	725	644	546
		0.3	804	703	638	559
		0.5	796	684	630	564
		0.8	771	644	602	562
		1.0	696	564	524	524
	#1-5	0.0	809	725	645	548
		0.3	804	703	639	561
		0.5	796	684	631	567
		0.8	771	644	604	565
		1.0	696	565	527	527
2. Separate assessment	#2-1	0.0	817	618	811	809
		0.3	812	603	806	804
		0.5	804	589	797	795
		0.8	777	559	769	769
		1.0	701	493	689	689
	#2-2	0.0	819	661	649	552
		0.3	814	654	643	565
		0.5	806	646	635	571
		0.8	780	622	608	569
		1.0	705	560	531	531
	#2-3	0.0	817	660	811	809
		0.3	811	653	805	803
		0.5	803	645	797	794
		0.8	776	620	770	767
		1.0	700	557	688	688
	#2-4	0.0	807	725	803	799
		0.3	801	702	796	793
		0.5	793	683	788	785
		0.8	767	643	761	758
		1.0	691	563	681	681

The efficacy and futility critical boundaries are determined commonly by the OF, using the Lan–DeMets error-spending method for the Type I and Type II errors with equally or unequally spaced increments of information

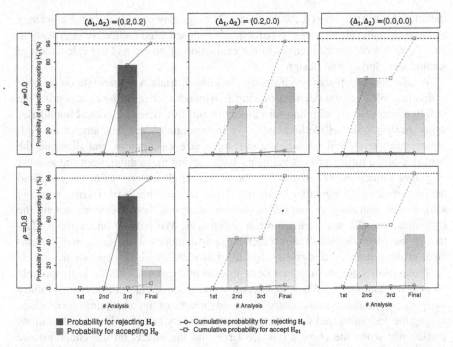

Fig. 4.2 The probability of rejecting or accepting H_0 when using Design #2-2 shown in Table 4.1, with $\rho_T = \rho_C = \rho = 0.0$ and 0.8, and $(\Delta_1, \Delta_2) = (0.2, 0.2), (0.0, 0.2)$ and $(0.0, 0.0)$. The efficacy and futility critical boundaries are determined commonly by the OF, using the Lan–DeMets error-spending method for the Type I and Type II errors with equally or unequally spaced increments of information

assessments at later interim analyses are conducted for both endpoints, the smallest MSS is given by Designs #2-4. The largest ASN reduction under $(\Delta_1, \Delta_2) = (0.2, 0.2)$ is given by Design #2-1, but the largest ASN reduction under $(\Delta_1, \Delta_2) = (0.0, 0.2)$ and $(0.0, 0.0)$ by #2-2.

Figure 4.2 summarizes the probability of rejecting or accepting H_0 when using Design #2-2 shown in Table 4.1, with $\rho = 0.0$ and 0.8, and $(\Delta_1, \Delta_2) = (0.2, 0.2), (0.0, 0.2)$ and $(0.0, 0.0)$. For $(\Delta_1, \Delta_2) = (0.2, 0.2)$ or $(0.0, 0.2)$, when $\rho = 0.0$, it is difficult to reject or accept H_0 at the earlier analyses, but easier later on. On the other hand, as ρ goes toward one, it is easier to reject or accept H_0 at the earlier analyses. For $(\Delta_1, \Delta_2) = (0.0, 0.0)$, it is easier to reject H_0 at the earlier analyses, but difficult later on.

4.4 Summary

Increasingly, clinical trials are being designed with more than one primary endpoint to more comprehensively evaluate intervention's multidimensional effects. As with trials involving a single primary endpoint, designing co-primary endpoint trials to include interim analyses (i.e., with repeated testing) may provide resource efficiency and minimize the number of trial participants exposed to an ineffective intervention. However, this creates challenges in the evaluation of power and the calculation of sample size during trial design.

We discuss group-sequential designs in clinical trials with multiple co-primary endpoints. We evaluate decision-making frameworks for rejecting or accepting the null hypothesis (early stopping for efficacy or futility), based on critical boundaries using group-sequential methodology. We incorporate correlations among the endpoints into the critical boundary and sample size calculations and illustrate the behavior of the futility critical boundary with varying mean differences and number of planned analyses. We investigate the operating characteristics of the proposed decision-making frameworks in terms of the power, the Type I error rate and sample size with varying number of planned analyses, the correlations among the endpoints, and the standardized mean differences. We provide an example illustrating the methods and discuss practical considerations when designing the efficient group-sequential designs in clinical trials with co-primary endpoints.

These results are useful when designing an efficient clinical trial with multiple co-primary endpoints. When conducting group-sequential efficacy and futility assessments in these trials, there is an advantage of incorporating correlations among the endpoints into the futility critical boundary and sample size calculations particularly when the correlations are large and the effects on the endpoints are similar. A larger number of planned analyses decrease the power, but increase the reduction in ASN. Efficacy and futility assessments at earlier information times increase the power but decrease the reduction in ASN. The power for assessing efficacy and futility at different interim analyses time-points is larger than simultaneous assessment. Careful consideration is needed regarding the frequency and timing of the futility and efficacy assessments. When only conducting futility assessments for either of the two endpoints at the first interim analysis and then only efficacy assessments for both endpoints at later interim analyses, power is not greatly affected by the magnitude of the standardized mean difference.

References

Ando Y, Hamasaki T, Evans SR, Asakura K, Sugimoto T, Sozu T, Ohno Y (2015) Sample size considerations in clinical trials when comparing two interventions using multiple co-primary binary relative risk contrasts. Stat Biopharm Res 7:81–94

Asakura K, Hamasaki T, Sugimoto T, Hayashi K, Evans SR, Sozu T (2014) Sample size determination in group-sequential clinical trials with two co-primary endpoints. Stat Med 33:2897–2913

Asakura K, Hamasaki T, Evans SR (2015) Interim evaluation of efficacy or futility in group-sequential clinical trials with multiple co-primary endpoints. The 2015 Joint Statistical Meetings, Seattle, USA, 8–13 August

Chang MN, Hwang IK, Shih WJ (1998) Group sequential designs using both Type I and Type II error probability spending functions. Commun Stat Theor Methods 27:1323–1339

Cheng Y, Ray S, Chang M, Menon S (2014) Statistical monitoring of clinical trials with multiple co-primary endpoints using multivariate B-value. Stat Biopharm Res 6:241–250

Chuang-Stein C, Stryszak P, Dmitrienko A, Offen W (2007) Challenge of multiple co-primary endpoints: a new approach. Stat Med 26:1181–1192

Cook RJ, Farewell VT (1994) Guideline for monitoring efficacy and toxicity responses in clinical trials. Biometrics 50s:1146–1162

DeMets DL, Ware JH (1980) Group sequential methods for clinical trials with a one-sided hypothesis. Biometrika 67:651–660

DeMets DL, Ware JH (1982) Asymmetric group sequential boundaries for monitoring clinical trials. Biometrika 69:661–663

Gould AL, Pecore VJ (1982) Group sequential methods for clinical trials allowing early acceptance of H_0 and incorporating costs. Biometrika 69:75–80

Green R, Schneider LS, Amato DA, Beelen AP, Wilcock G, Swabb EA, Zavitz KH, for the Tarenflurbil Phase 3 Study Group (2009) Effect of tarenflurbil on cognitive decline and activities of daily living in patients with mild Alzheimer disease: a randomized controlled trial. J Am Med Assoc 302:2557–2564

Hamasaki T, Asakura K, Evans SR, Sugimoto T, Sozu T (2015) Group-sequential strategies in clinical trials with multiple co-primary outcomes. Stat Biopharm Res 7:36–54

Jennison C, Turnbull BW (1993) Group sequential tests for bivariate response: interim analyses of clinical trials with both efficacy and safety. Biometrics 49:741–752

Kordzakhia G, Siddiqui O, Huque MF (2010) Method of balanced adjustment in testing co-primary endpoints. Stat Med 29:2055–2066

Lachin JM (2005) A review of methods for futility stopping based on conditional power. Stat Med 24:2747–2764

Lan KKG, DeMets DL (1983) Discrete sequential boundaries for clinical trials. Biometrika 70:659–663

Lan KKG, Simon R, Halperin M (1982) Stochastically curtailed tests in long-term clinical trials. Commun Stat Theor Methods 1:207–219

O'Brien PC, Fleming TR (1979) A multiple testing procedure for clinical trials. Biometrics 35:549–556

Pharmaceuticals and Medical Devices Agency (2010a) Review report of memantine. 1 Dec 2010, Pharmaceuticals and Medical Devices Agency, Tokyo (in Japanese). Available at: http://www.pmda.go.jp/drugs/2011/P201100018/43057400_22300AMX00423_A100_2.pdf. Accessed 25 Nov 2015

Pharmaceuticals and Medical Devices Agency (2010b) Review report of galantamine hydrobromide. 1 Dec 2010, Pharmaceuticals and Medical Devices Agency, Tokyo (in Japanese). Available at: http://www.pmda.go.jp/drugs/2011/P201100024/80015500_23000AMX00426_A100_1.pdf. Accessed 25 Nov 2015

Pharmaceuticals and Medical Devices Agency (2011) Review report of rivastigmine. 11 March 2011, Pharmaceuticals and Medical Devices Agency, Tokyo (in Japanese). Available at: http://www.pmda.go.jp/drugs/2011/P201100075/18018800_22300AMX00529000_A100_1.pdf. Accessed 25 Nov 2015

Snapinn S, Chen MG, Jiang Q, Koutsoukos T (2006) Assessment of futility in clinical trials. Pharm Stat 5:273–281

Ware JH, Muller JE, Braunwald E (1985) The futility index: an approach to the cost-effective termination of randomized clinical trials. Am J Med 78:635–643

Whitehead J, Matsushita T (2003) Stopping clinical trials because of treatment ineffectiveness: a comparison of a futility design with a method of stochastic curtailment. Stat Med 22:677–687

Chapter 5
Interim Evaluation of Efficacy in Clinical Trials with Two Primary Endpoints

Abstract In this chapter, we provide an overview of the fundamental concepts and technical details for group-sequential designs for clinical trials comparing two interventions based on two primary endpoints. In this situation, there are many procedures for controlling the Type I error rate. We discuss the simplest procedure, i.e., the weighted Bonferroni procedure which is commonly applied in practice. We evaluate the behavior of the sample size, power, and Type I error rate associated with the procedure.

Keywords Average sample size · Efficacy stopping · Lan–DeMets error-spending method · Maximum sample size · Recycled significance level · Union–intersection test · Weighted Bonferroni procedure

5.1 Introduction

In the previous chapters, we discuss group-sequential methods in clinical trial with two co-primary endpoints. In this chapter, we discuss group-sequential designs for trails with two primary endpoints, i.e., where the trial is designed to evaluate whether the intervention is superior to the control on *at least one* of the endpoints.

In clinical trials with two primary endpoints, adjustments must be made to control the Type I error rate. There are many procedures for controlling the Type I error rate [e.g., see Bretz et al. (2011), Dmitrienko et al. (2010), and Wiens and Dmitrienko (2010)]. When the aim was to evaluate an effect on at least one endpoint (multiple primary endpoints), Tang and Geller (1999), Glimm et al. (2010), and Tamhane et al. (2010, 2012) considered methods based on the closed testing principle, and Kosorok et al. (2004) discussed a global alpha-spending function to control the Type I error and a multiple decision rule to control error rates for concluding wrong alternative hypotheses. For group-sequential designs with other inferential goal settings, Pocock et al. (1987) and Tang et al. (1989) discussed a method based on a generalized least squares procedure by O'Brien (1984), and Jennison and Turnbull (1991) discuss a method based on chi-square and *F* test

T. Hamasaki et al., *Group-Sequential Clinical Trials with Multiple Co-Objectives*, JSS Research Series in Statistics, DOI 10.1007/978-4-431-55900-9_5

statistics, where the trial is designed if the test intervention has an overall effect across the endpoints compared with the control intervention, but does not necessarily evaluate the effect on any specific endpoint. For more details, see Jennison and Turnbull (2000).

In this chapter, we discuss the weighted Bonferroni procedure which is well-known and widely utilized in practice. When considering the weighted Bonferroni procedure, we assume that both outcomes are equally important and an ordering of the outcomes is not prespecified for hypothesis testing. We evaluate the behavior of the power, Type I error rate, and the sample size associated with the procedure.

5.2   Decision-Making Frameworks and Stopping Rules

5.2.1   Notation and Statistical Setting

Similarly to Sect. 2.2, consider a randomized, group-sequential clinical trial comparing the test intervention (T) with the control intervention (C). Two continuous outcomes, EP1 and EP2, are to be evaluated as primary endpoints (i.e., $K = 2$). Suppose that a maximum of L analyses is planned, where the same number of planned analyses with the same information space is selected for both endpoints. Suppose that the trial is designed to evaluate EP1 and EP2 as primary endpoints, i.e. , if T is superior to C on at least one of EP1 and EP2.

Let n_l and $r_C n_l$ be the cumulative number of participants on the T and the C at the lth analysis ($l = 1, \ldots, L$), respectively, where r_C is the allocation ratio of the C to the T. Hence, up to n_L and $r_C n_L$ participants are recruited and randomly assigned to the T and the C, respectively. Then, there are n_L paired outcomes (Y_{T1i}, Y_{T2i}) ($i = 1, \ldots, n_L$) for the T and $r_C n_L$ paired outcomes (Y_{C1j}, Y_{C2j}) ($j = 1, \ldots, r_C n_L$) for the C. Assume that (Y_{T1i}, Y_{T2i}) and (Y_{C1j}, Y_{C2j}) are independently bivariate distributed with mean $E[Y_{Tki}] = \mu_{Tk}$ and $E[Y_{Ckj}] = \mu_{Ck}$, variances $var[Y_{Tki}] = \sigma_{Tk}^2$ and $var[Y_{Ckj}] = \sigma_{Ck}^2$, and correlation $corr[Y_{T1i}, Y_{T2i}] = \rho_T$ and $corr[Y_{C1j}, Y_{C2j}] = \rho_C$, respectively ($k = 1, 2$). For simplicity, the variances are assumed to be known and common, i.e., $\sigma_{Tk}^2 = \sigma_{Ck}^2 = \sigma_k^2$, similarly as in the previous chapters.

Let $\delta_k = \mu_{Tk} - \mu_{Ck}$ and $\Delta_k = \delta_k / \sigma_k (k = 1, 2)$ denote the mean differences and standardized mean differences for the T and the C, respectively. Suppose that positive values of δ_k represent a benefit for the T. There is an interest in conducting a hypothesis test to evaluate whether the T is superior to the C on at least one endpoint in a group-sequential setting. The null hypothesis H_0: $H_{01} \cap H_{02}$ versus the alternative hypothesis H_1: $H_{11} \cup H_{12}$ is tested at the significance level of α [union–intersection test: Berger (1982)], where the hypotheses for each endpoint are H_{0k}: $\delta_k \leq 0$ versus H_{1k}: $\delta_k > 0$ (test the intersection H_0 of both individual nulls against the union alternative H_1). This hypothesis is tested based on the test statistics (Z_{1l}, Z_{2l}), which are the same statistics defined in Sect. 2.2. In contrast to multiple co-primary endpoints, the Type I error rate needs to be controlled adequately since the Type I error rate increases as the number of endpoints to be evaluated increases.

5.2.2 Weighted Bonferroni Procedure

The weighted Bonferroni procedure is the simplest p-value-based procedure. The procedure distributes the overall α between the two endpoints with the positive weight w_k (>0), and each endpoint is tested at $\alpha_k = w_k \alpha$ ($k = 1, 2$), where $w_1 + w_2 = 1$. A decision-making framework associated with hypothesis testing based on the weighted Bonferroni procedure is very simple. It is to reject H_0 if statistical significance of T relative to C is achieved for at least one endpoint at any interim time point until the final analysis. The stopping rule is formally given as follows:

At the lth analysis ($l = 1, \ldots, L - 1$)

if $Z_{1l} > c_{1l}^E(\alpha_1)$ or $Z_{2l} > c_{2l}^E(\alpha_2)$, then reject H_0 and stop the trial, otherwise, continue to the ($l + 1$) th analysis,

at the Lth analysis

if $Z_{1L} > c_{1L}^E(\alpha_1)$ or $Z_{2L} > c_{2L}^E(\alpha_2)$, then reject H_0, otherwise, do not reject H_0,

where $c_{1l}^E(\alpha_1)$ and $c_{2l}^E(\alpha_2)$ are the critical boundaries. Similarly as in multiple co-primary endpoints discussed in Chap. 2, the critical boundaries are constant and selected separately, using any group-sequential method to control the overall Type I error rate, as if they were a single primary endpoint, without regard to the other primary endpoint. For example, consider a group-sequential clinical trial with five planned analyses ($L = 5$). The (unweighted) Bonferroni procedure is applied to allocate $\alpha = 2.5$ % between the two endpoints with equal weight ($w_1 = w_2 = 0.5$) and the hypothesis for each endpoint is tested at the significance level of $\alpha_1 = \alpha_2 = 1.25$ %. If the critical boundaries for both endpoints are determined by the O'Brien–Fleming-type boundary (OF) (O'Brien and Fleming 1979), using the Lan–DeMets error-spending method (Lan and DeMets 1984), with equally-spaced increments of information, then the critical boundaries for each analysis are 5.4633, 3.7803, 3.0270, 2.5879, and 2.2959. Figure 5.1 shows the rejection region for the null hypothesis with the number of planned analyses. For example, if the test statistic for EP1 is larger than the critical boundary of 2.5879 at the fourth analysis (but the test statistic for EP2 is smaller than the critical boundary), then H_0 is rejected and the trial is terminated. If the test statistics for both endpoints are smaller

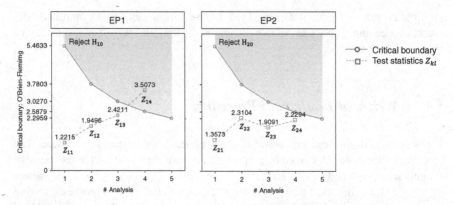

Fig. 5.1 The region for rejecting the null hypothesis in a group-sequential clinical trial with five planned analyses ($L = 5$). The Bonferroni procedure is applied to allocate $\alpha = 2.5$ % between the two endpoints with equal weight ($w_1 = w_2 = 0.5$) and the hypothesis for each endpoint is tested at the significance level of $\alpha_1 = \alpha_2 = 1.25$ % for a one-sided test. The critical boundaries for both endpoints are determined by the OF, using the Lan–DeMets error-spending method with equally spaced increments of information

than the critical boundary, then H_0 is not rejected and the subsequent hypothesis testing is repeatedly conducted for both outcomes until superiority is demonstrated on at least one endpoint or the trial is completed.

The corresponding power for detecting the effect on the least one endpoint is given as follows:

$$1 - \beta = \Pr\left[\left\{\bigcup_{l=1}^{L} A_{1l}\right\} \bigcup \left\{\bigcup_{l=1}^{L} A_{2l}\right\} \middle| H_1\right], \tag{5.1}$$

where $A_{kl} = \{Z_{kl} > c_{kl}^{E}(\alpha_k)\}$.

As described in Sect. 2.2.3, we calculate two sample sizes, i.e., the maximum sample size (MSS) and the average sample number (ASN) (i.e., expected sample size) based on the power (5.1). Recall that the MSS is the sample size required for the final analysis to achieve the desired power $1 - \beta$. The ASN is the expected sample size under hypothetical reference values and provides information regarding the number of participants anticipated in a group-sequential clinical trial in order to reach a decision point.

Figure 5.2 illustrates the behavior of the power for detecting the effect on at least one outcome for varying correlations ($\rho_T = \rho_C = \rho$), weight, and critical boundary combinations for a given sample size in a group-sequential clinical trial with $L = 2$, assuming equal standardized mean differences $\Delta_1 = \Delta_2 = 0.2$. The sample size of 393 per intervention group (equally sized groups) has 80 % power to detect a standardized mean difference for each outcome at the (unadjusted) 2.5 % significance level for a one-sided test. The weighted Bonferroni procedure is applied to allocate $\alpha = 2.5$ % between the two endpoints with the weight w_k, and the

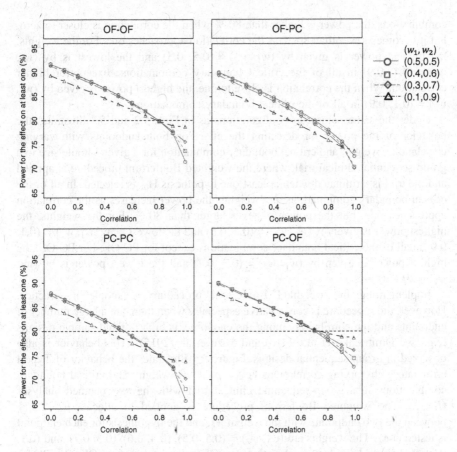

Fig. 5.2 Behavior of the power for detecting an effect on the least endpoint for varying correlations, weight, and critical boundary combinations for a given sample size in a group-sequential clinical trial with the two planned analyses ($L = 2$), assuming equal standardized mean differences $\Delta_1 = \Delta_2 = 0.2$. The sample size of 393 per intervention group (equally sized groups) has 80 % power to detect a standardized mean difference for each endpoint at the (unadjusted) 2.5 % significance level for a one-sided test. The weighted Bonferroni procedure is applied to allocate $\alpha = 2.5$ % between the two endpoints with the weight w_k, and the hypothesis for each endpoint is tested at α_k. The weights are $(w_1, w_2) = (0.5, 0.5)$, $(0.4, 0.6)$, $(0.3, 0.7)$, and $(0.1, 0.9)$; the critical boundary combinations are OF for both endpoints (OF-OF), PC for both endpoints (PC-PC), OF for EP1 and PC for EP2 (OF-PC), and PC for EP1 and OF for EP2 (PC-OF)

hypothesis for each endpoint is tested at α_k. The weights are $(w_1, w_2) = (0.5, 0.5)$, $(0.4, 0.6)$, $(0.3, 0.7)$, and $(0.1, 0.9)$; the critical boundary combinations are the OF for both endpoints (OF-OF), the Pocock-type boundary (PC) (Pocock 1977) for both endpoints (PC-PC), OF for EP1 and PC for EP2 (OF-PC), PC for EP1 and OF for EP2 (OF-PC).

Similarly as in fixed-sample designs shown in Senn and Bretz (2007) and Sozu et al. (2015), the figure shows that in all of the weights and the critical boundary combinations, the power is higher than 80 % when the correlation is closer to zero, but it becomes lower than 80 % as the correlation approaches one. For the weights, the highest power is given by $(w_1, w_2) = (0.5, 0.5)$ and the lowest is by $(w_1, w_2) = (0.1, 0.9)$ in all of the critical boundary combinations, except for higher correlation. When the correlation is close to one, the highest power is given by $(w_1, w_2) = (0.1, 0.9)$ in all of the critical boundary combinations.

Under the same parameter configurations as in Figs. 5.2 and 5.3 illustrates the behavior of the power for detecting the effect on both endpoints with varying correlations, weight, and critical boundary combination for a given sample size in a group-sequential clinical trial, where the weighted Bonferroni procedure is applied and the trial is terminated when at least one hypothesis H_{0k} is rejected. In all of the critical boundary combinations and weights, the power increases as the correlation approaches one, but the power is never larger than 80 %. For the weights, the highest power is given by $(w_1, w_2) = (0.5, 0.5)$ and the lowest is by $(w_1, w_2) = (0.1, 0.9)$ in all of the critical boundary combinations except for PC-OF. For PC-OF, the highest power is given by $(w_1, w_2) = (0.3, 0.7)$ and the lowest power is by $(w_1, w_2) = (0.1, 0.9)$.

Implementing the weighted Bonferroni procedure is simple in practice. However, the procedure is conservative especially when there are a large number of endpoints and the correlation among the endpoints is high in fixed-sample designs [e.g., see Dmitrienko et al. (2010) and Sozu et al. (2015)]. This behavior is also observed in group-sequential designs. Figure 5.4 illustrates the behavior of Type I error rate with varying correlations ($\rho_T = \rho_C = \rho$), weight, and critical boundary combinations in a group-sequential clinical trial with the two planned analyses ($L = 2$). The weighted Bonferroni procedure is applied to allocate $\alpha = 2.5$ % between the two endpoints with the weight w_k, and the hypothesis for each endpoint is tested at α_k. The weights are $(w_1, w_2) = (0.5, 0.5), (0.4, 0.6), (0.3, 0.7)$, and $(0.1, 0.9)$; the critical boundary combinations are OF for both endpoints (OF-OF), PC for both endpoints (PC-PC), OF for EP1 and PC for EP2 (OF-PC), and PC for EP1 and OF for EP2 (PC-OF). The Type I error rate is below the nominal error rate when the endpoints are positively and highly correlated. An appropriate choice of the weight could lead to improve Type I error and an increase in the power. As Wiens and Dmitrienko (2010) suggest, one strategy is to determine the weight corresponding directly to the size of the mean difference to maximize the probability that at least one hypothesis is rejected or to maintain similar power for each endpoint.

5.2.3 Weighted Bonferroni Procedure with the Reallocated Significance Level

As shown in Fig. 5.3, the power for detecting a joint effect on both endpoints based on the weighted Bonferroni procedure is modest, especially when the correlation between the endpoints is small. By using the idea of reallocating the significance

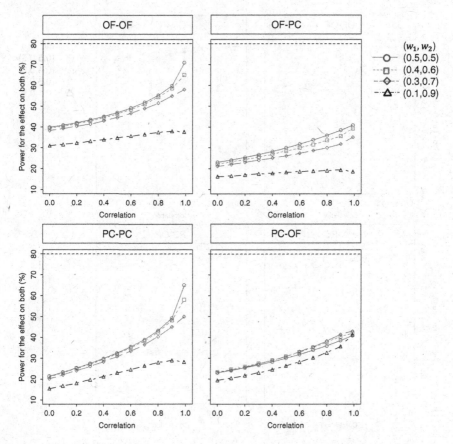

Fig. 5.3 Behavior of the power for detecting an effect on both endpoints (under the sample size when the at least one hypothesis is rejected and the trial is stopped) for varying correlations, weight, and critical boundary combinations for a given sample size in a group-sequential clinical trial with the two planned analyses ($L = 2$), assuming equal standardized mean differences $\Delta_1 = \Delta_2 = 0.2$. The sample size of 393 per intervention group (equally sized groups) has 80 % power to detect a standardized mean difference for each endpoint at the (unadjusted) 2.5 % significance level for a one-sided test. The weighted Bonferroni procedure is applied to allocate $\alpha = 2.5$ % between the two endpoints with the weight w_k, and the hypothesis for each endpoint is tested at α_k. The weights are $(w_1, w_2) = (0.5, 0.5)$, $(0.4, 0.6)$, $(0.3, 0.7)$, and $(0.1, 0.9)$; the critical boundary combinations are OF for both endpoints (OF-OF), PC for both endpoints (PC-PC), OF for EP1 and PC for EP2 (OF-PC), and PC for EP1 and OF for EP2 (PC-PC)

levels discussed in Bretz et al. (2009) and Burman et al. (2009), a more powerful Bonferroni procedure can be constructed in a group-sequential clinical trial with multiple primary endpoints (Maurer and Bretz 2013; Ye et al. 2013; Xi and Tamhane 2015).

The concept of reallocating the significance level is simple. When considering a clinical trial with two primary endpoints, the significance level from the rejected

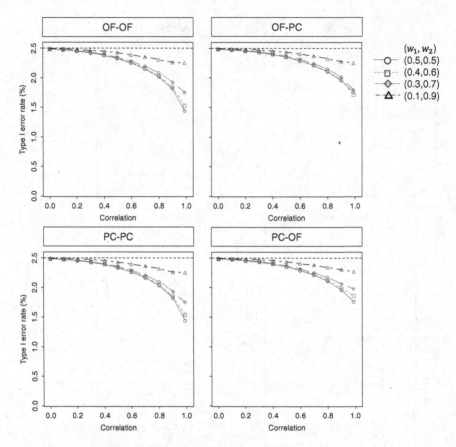

Fig. 5.4 Behavior of Type I error rate with varying correlations, weight, and critical boundary combinations in a group-sequential clinical trial with the two planned analyses ($L = 2$). The Bonferroni procedure is applied to allocate $\alpha = 2.5\ \%$ between the two endpoints with the weight w_k, and the hypothesis for each endpoint is tested at α_k. The weights are $(w_1, w_2) = (0.5, 0.5)$, $(0.4, 0.6)$, $(0.3, 0.7)$, and $(0.1, 0.9)$; the critical boundary combinations are OF for both endpoints (OF-OF), PC for both endpoints (PC-PC), OF for EP1 and PC for EP2 (OF-PC), and PC for EP1 and OF for EP2 (PC-OF)

hypothesis for one endpoint is reallocated to the not-yet-rejected hypothesis for other endpoint. However, in a group-sequential setting, one must decide how to reallocate the significance level to the interim analyses for the not-yet-rejected hypothesis for other endpoint (Xi and Tamhane 2015). When applying the Bonferroni–Holm procedure in a group-sequential clinical trial with two primary endpoints, Ye et al. (2013) consider two methods for reallocating the significance level: (i) reallocate the significance level from the rejected hypothesis for one endpoint to all analyses (including the already-passed and not-yet-passed interims, and the final analysis) for the not-yet-rejected hypothesis for the other endpoint, and (ii) reallocate the significance level from the rejected hypothesis for one endpoint to the final analysis for the not-yet-rejected hypothesis for the other endpoint. There is a loss of reallocating the significance level as the significance level is reallocated to already-passed interims in the former method (Xi and Tamhan 2015). The latter has no such loss in the significance level although the trial may continue to the final analysis. Xi and Tamhane (2015) discuss methods of reallocating the significance level from the rejected hypothesis for one endpoint to the later interims from a specified interim. In these methods, if the full significance level for the rejected hypothesis for one endpoint is reallocated to the not-yet-rejected hypothesis for other endpoint, then the Type I error rate for rejecting H_0 is inflated over the prespecified significance level, depending on the correlation and standardized mean difference (Hung et al. 2007; Glimm et al. 2009; Xi and Tamhane 2015).

Although there are several ways to reallocate the significance level, we here consider the idea in Ye et al. (2013) where the significance level is the full significance level from the rejected hypothesis for one endpoint and it is reallocated to all of the analyses for other endpoint, including to already-passed interims. However, at the subsequent analyses, the hypothesis for the other endpoint is tested using the updated critical boundaries based on the originally allocated and reallocated significance levels although the critical boundaries at already-passed interims are not updated. So that, first we can calculate the two sets of critical boundaries: one is based on α_k and the other is based on $\alpha = \alpha_1 + \alpha_2$, not necessarily calculating how much the significance level has been already spent and updating the critical boundaries based on the originally allocated and reallocated significance levels. For example, consider a clinical trial with a maximum number of planned analyses $L = 5$ and equally spaced increments of information, and the OF is used to reject the null hypothesis for both endpoints EP1 and EP2 at the significance level of $\alpha_1 = \alpha_2 = 1.25$ % for a one-sided test based on an unweighted Bonferroni procedure. The critical boundaries for each analysis are 5.4633, 3.7803, 3.0270, 2.5879, and 2.2959 based on $\alpha_k = 1.25$ %, and 4.8769, 3.3569, 2.6803, 2.2898, and 2.0310 based on $\alpha = 2.5$ %, respectively. If the test statistic for EP1 is larger than the critical boundary of 2.5879 at the fourth analysis (but the test statistic for EP2 is smaller than the critical boundary), then the hypothesis test for EP2 is tested again with 2.2898 at the fourth analysis and with 2.0310 at the final analysis.

Under the same parameter settings and configurations as in Figs. 5.3 and 5.5 displays the behavior of the power for detecting the effect on both endpoints with varying correlations, weight, and critical boundary combination for a given sample size in a group-sequential clinical trial, where the weighted Bonferroni procedure with reallocating the significance level is applied and the trial is terminated when at least one hypothesis H_{0k} is rejected. Comparing Fig. 5.5 with Fig. 5.3, the power is much improved by using the weighted Bonferroni procedure with reallocating the significance level except for OF-OF and $(w_1, w_2) = (0.4, 0.6)$ or $(0.3, 0.7)$. In all of the critical boundary combinations and weights, the power increases as the correlation approaches one, especially in PC-PC and PC-OF, the power is larger than 80 % with large correlation. For the weights, the highest power is given by $(w_1, w_2) = (0.5, 0.5)$ and the lowest is by $(w_1, w_2) = (0.4, 0.6)$ in all of the critical boundary combinations.

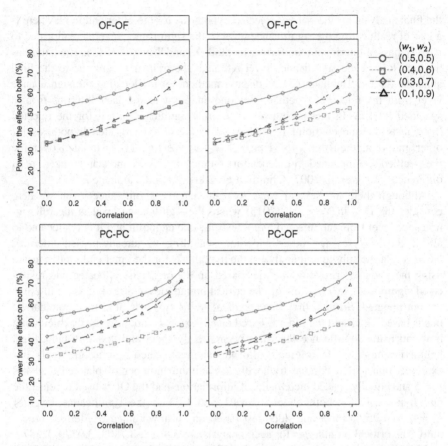

Fig. 5.5 Behavior of the power for detecting the effect on both endpoints with varying correlations, weighting, and critical boundary combinations for a given sample size in a group-sequential clinical trial with the two planned analyses ($L = 2$), assuming equal standardized mean differences $\Delta_1 = \Delta_2 = 0.2$. The sample size of 393 per intervention group (equally sized groups) has 80 % power to detect a standardized mean difference for each endpoint at the (unadjusted) 2.5 % significance level for a one-sided test. In addition, the weighted Bonferroni procedure with reallocating the significance level is applied and the trial is terminated when at least one hypothesis H_{k0} is rejected. The weights are $(w_1, w_2) = (0.5, 0.5), (0.4, 0.6), (0.3, 0.7)$, and $(0.1, 0.9)$; the critical boundary combinations are OF for both endpoints (OF-OF), PC for both endpoints (PC-PC), OF for EP1 and PC for EP2 (OF-PC), and PC for EP1 and OF for EP2 (PC-OF)

5.3   Illustration

Table 5.1 displays the MSS and ASN per intervention group in a group-sequential clinical trial with the two planned analyses ($L = 2$), assuming equal standardized mean differences ($\Delta_1 = \Delta_2 = 0.2$). The MSS is calculated to detect the effect on at least one endpoint with 80 % power at 2.5 % significance level for a one-sided test.

Table 5.1 MSS and ASN per intervention group (equally sized groups) in a group-sequential clinical trial with $L = 2$, assuming equal standardized mean differences $\Delta_1 = \Delta_2 = 0.2$

Weight (w_1, w_2)	Critical boundary combination	Correlation ρ	Without reallocating			With reallocating		
			MSS	ASN (H_1)	Power2	Power2	Power diff	
(0.50, 0.50)	OF-OF	0.0	283	270	25.8	37.0	11.2
		0.3	317	300	34.4	46.2	11.8
		0.5	343	323	41.1	53.3	12.2
		0.8	394	369	55.3	67.3	12.1
	PC-PC	0.0	322	248	15.4	25.7	10.3
		0.3	358	274	24.2	36.4	12.2
		0.5	386	295	31.8	44.9	13.2
		0.8	441	337	48.4	62.2	13.9
	OF-PC	0.0	301	258	15.9	25.6	9.7
		0.3	335	283	22.1	33.5	12.4
		0.5	362	303	27.4	39.9	11.3
		0.8	412	339	37.5	51.6	14.0
(0.75, 0.25)	OF-OF	0.0	290	276	24.4	38.3	13.9
		0.3	323	305	32.2	47.3	15.0
		0.5	349	327	38.3	54.3	16.0
		0.8	395	368	49.6	67.4	17.8
	PC-PC	0.0	330	254	14.5	27.5	13.0
		0.3	365	279	22.6	38.1	15.5
		0.5	392	299	29.5	46.5	17.0
		0.8	442	337	43.4	63.0	19.6
	OF-PC	0.0	306	268	15.5	29.1	13.6
		0.3	339	294	22.1	37.6	15.4
		0.5	362	312	27.6	44.1	16.5
		0.8	403	347	39.0	56.7	17.7
	PC-OF	0.0	312	261	14.8	25.4	10.6
		0.3	346	285	19.7	32.7	13.0
		0.5	373	303	23.5	38.5	15.0
		0.8	423	335	29.7	48.7	18.9
(0.99, 0.01)	OF-OF	0.0	350	326	12.4	48.0	35.6
		0.3	371	343	14.9	54.2	39.3
		0.5	383	353	15.9	58.8	42.9
		0.8	395	363	15.7	67.1	51.5
	PC-PC	0.0	394	303	7.0	40.3	33.4
		0.3	416	318	9.6	48.8	39.1
		0.5	429	327	11.1	54.8	43.7
		0.8	442	337	11.5	64.9	53.4
	OF-PC	0.0	359	327	8.2	45.3	37.1

(continued)

Table 5.1 (continued)

Weight (w_1, w_2)	Critical boundary combination	Correlation ρ	Without reallocating			With reallocating	
			MSS	ASN (H_1)	Power2	Power2	Power diff
		0.3	377	342	10.9	52.6	41.8
		0.5	387	352	12.6	58.0	45.4
		0.8	395	361	14.6	67.0	52.4
	PC-OF	0.0	382	302	7.6	31.7	24.1
		0.3	407	317	8.6	37.4	28.7
		0.5	423	326	8.8	41.4	32.7
		0.8	440	336	7.6	47.8	40.2

The MSS is calculated to detect the effect on at least one endpoint with 80 % power at 2.5 % significance level for a one-sided test. The weighted Bonferroni procedure with/without the reallocated significance level is applied with the weight (w_1, w_2), and the hypothesis for each endpoint is tested at $\alpha_k = w_k\alpha$. The weights are (w_1, w_2) = (0.5, 0.5), (0.75, 0.25), and (0.99, 0.01). The critical boundary is determined by using Lan–DeMets error-spending method and the critical boundary combinations are OF for both endpoints (OF-OF), PC for both endpoints (PC-PC), OF for EP1 and PC for EP2 (OF-PC), PC for EP1 and OF for EP2 (PC-OF). The ASN is calculated under H_1. The power for detecting a joint effect on both endpoints (Power2) is calculated under the given MSS. Furthermore, the difference in power with vs. without the reallocated significance level is provided (Power diff)

The weighted Bonferroni procedure with/without the reallocated significance level is applied to the weights (w_1, w_2), and the hypothesis for each endpoint is tested at $\alpha_k = w_k\alpha$. The weights are (w_1, w_2) = (0.5, 0.5), (0.75, 0.25), and (0.99, 0.01). The critical boundary is determined by using Lan–DeMets error-spending method and the critical boundary combinations are OF for both endpoints (OF-OF), PC for both endpoints (PC-PC), OF for EP1 and PC for EP2 (OF-PC), and PC for EP1 and OF for EP2 (PC-OF). The ASN is calculated under H_1. The power for detecting a joint effect on both endpoints (Power2) is calculated under the given MSS.

When applying the weighted Bonferroni procedure without the reallocated significance level, the MSS increases with increasing correlation in all of the critical boundary combinations and weights. The largest MSS is observed in PC-OF with (w_1, w_2) = (0.99, 0.01) and $\rho_T = \rho_C = \rho = 0.8$, and the smallest is in OF-OF with (w_1, w_2) = (0.50, 0.50) and $\rho = 0.0$. The largest reduction of 17.4 % in sample size of ASN to MSS is observed in PC-PC with (w_1, w_2) = (0.99, 0.01) and $\rho = 0.0$, and the smallest of 1.2 % is observed in OF-OF with (w_1, w_2) = (0.50, 0.50) or (0.75, 0.25) with $\rho = 0.0$.

Using weighted Bonferroni with the reallocated significance level increases the power for detecting the joint effect on both endpoints, compared with the option of not using the reallocated significance level. In all of the critical boundary combinations and weights, the absolute improvement increases as the correlation approaches one. The maximum absolute improvement of 53.4 % is observed in the case of PC-PC with (w_1, w_2) = (0.99, 0.01) and $\rho = 0.8$, and the minimum of 9.7 % is observed in the case of OF-PC with (w_1, w_2) = (0.5, 0.5) and $\rho = 0.0$.

5.4 Summary

We provide an overview of the concepts and technical fundamentals regarding group-sequential designs for clinical trials comparing two interventions with two primary endpoints. Without proper adjustments, the Type I error rate increases as the number of primary endpoints increases. There are many procedures that can be implemented for controlling the Type I error rate. We discuss a common procedure and simple procedure, i.e., the weighted Bonferroni procedure. We evaluate the behavior of the sample size, power, and Type I error rate associated with the Bonferroni procedure.

The behaviors of power and sample size for evaluating superiority for *at least one* endpoint with weighted Bonferroni procedure are very different from those for evaluating superiority for *all* endpoints discussed in Chap. 2 (multiple co-primary endpoints). The conservative sample size strategy when evaluating superiority for co-primary endpoints is to assume zero correlations among the endpoints if the two endpoints are known to be positively correlated. However, when evaluating superiority for at least one endpoint, assuming a correlation of one between endpoints is conservative. Thus, when considering multiple endpoints in clinical trials, it is important to distinguish between the two objectives, i.e., whether the trial is aiming to evaluate superiority of a test intervention relative to a control intervention on *all* primary endpoints or *at least one* primary endpoint.

References

Berger RL (1982) Multiparameter hypothesis testing and acceptance sampling. Technometrics 24:295–300

Bretz F, Maurer W, Brannath W, Posch M (2009) A graphical approach to sequentially rejective multiple test procedures. Stat Med 28:586–604

Bretz F, Hothorn T, Westfall P (2011) Multiple comparisons using R. Chapman and Hall, CRC Press, Boca Raton

Burman CF, Sonesson C, Guilbaud O (2009) A recycling framework for the construction of Bonferroni-based multiple tests. Stat Med 28:739–761

Dmitrienko A, Tamhane AC, Bretz F (2010) Multiple testing problems in pharmaceutical statistics. Chapman and Hall, CRC Press, Boca Raton

Glimm E, Mauer W, Bretz F (2009) Hierarchical testing of multiple endpoints in group-sequential trials. Stat Med 29:219–228

Glimm E, Mauer W, Bretz F (2010) Hierarchical testing of multiple endpoints in group-sequential trials. Stat Med 29:219–228

Hung HMJ, Wang SJ, O'Neill RT (2007) Statistical considerations for testing multiple endpoints in group sequential or adaptive clinical trials. J Biopharm Stat 17:1201–1210

Jennison C, Turnbull BW (1991) Exact calculations for sequential t, χ^2 and F tests. Biometrika 78:133–141

Jennison C, Turnbull BW (2000) Group sequential methods with applications to clinical trials. Chapman and Hall, CRC Press, Boca Raton

Kosorok MR, Shi Y, DeMets DL (2004) Design and analysis of group-sequential clinical trials with multiple primary endpoints. Biometrics 60:134–145

Lan KKG, DeMets DL (1984) Discrete sequential boundaries for clinical trials. Biometrika 70:659–663

Maurer W, Bretz F (2013) Multiple testing in group sequential trials using graphical approaches. Stat Biopharm Res 5:311–320

O'Brien PC (1984) Procedures for comparing samples with multiple endpoints. Biometrics 40:1079–1087

O'Brien PC, Fleming TR (1979) A multiple testing procedure for clinical trials. Biometrics 35:549–556

Pocock SJ (1977) Group sequential methods in the design and analysis of clinical trials. Biometrika 64:191–199

Pocock SJ, Geller NL, Tsiatis AA (1987) The analysis of multiple endpoints in clinical trials. Biometrics 43:487–498

Senn S, Bretz F (2007) Power and sample size when multiple endpoints are considered. Pharm Stat 6:161–170

Sozu T, Sugimoto T, Hamasaki T, Evans SR (2015) Sample size determination in clinical trials with multiple endpoints. Springer International Press, Cham

Tamhane AC, Mehta CR, Liu L (2010) Testing a primary and secondary endpoint in a group sequential design. Biometrics 66:1174–1184

Tamhane AC, Wu Y, Mehta C (2012) Adaptive extensions of a two-stage group sequential procedure for testing primary and secondary endpoints (I): unknown correlation between the endpoints. Stat Med 31:2027–2040

Tang DI, Geller NL (1999) Closed testing procedures for group sequential clinical trials with multiple endpoints. Biometrics 55:1188–1192

Tang DI, Gnecco C, Geller NL (1989) Design of group sequential clinical trials with multiple endpoints. J Am Stat Assoc 84:776–779

Wiens BL, Dmitrienko A (2010) On selecting a multiple comparison procedure for analysis of a clinical trial: fallback, fixed sequence, and related procedures. Stat Biopharm Res 2:22–32

Xi D, Tamhane AC (2015) Allocating recycled significance levels in group sequential procedures for multiple endpoints. Biometrical J 57:90–107

Ye Y, Li A, Lui L, Yao B (2013) A group sequential Holm procedure with multiple primary endpoints. Stat Med 32:1112–1124

Chapter 6
Group-Sequential Three-Arm Non-inferiority Clinical Trials

Abstract We discuss group-sequential three-arm non-inferiority (NI) clinical trials, i.e., trials that include a test intervention as well as active and placebo controls for evaluating both assay sensitivity and NI. We extend two existing approaches, the fixed margin and fraction approaches, to a group-sequential setting with two decision-making frameworks. We provide an example to illustrate the methods.

Keywords Assay sensitivity · Average sample number · Constancy · Fixed margin approach · Fraction approach · Maximum sample size · Non-inferiority · Type I error

6.1 Introduction

Active-controlled non-inferiority (NI) trial designs are an alternative to placebo-controlled superiority designs when a use of the placebo control is ethically undesirable due to the availability of a proven effective medical intervention. Active-controlled NI trial designs include an existing effective intervention such as an effective standard of care. In contrast to superiority trials where there is interest in evaluating whether an intervention is superior to a control (e.g., placebo), NI trials evaluate whether an intervention is non-inferior to the control. In a NI trial, the null hypothesis of inferiority is assumed to be true unless there are sufficient data to reject it in favor of the alternative (NI). NI is assessed by evaluating whether inferiority of a prespecified magnitude (called a NI margin) can be ruled out with reasonable confidence using confidence intervals. The NI margin is carefully selected to ensure that a NI result would (1) imply retention of the some of the effect that the active control has historically displayed (i.e., when compared to placebo) and (2) rule out clinically important levels of inferiority so that clinical application would be ethical and clinically acceptable.

For example, EMERALD 1 (conducted in the USA) and EMERALD 2 (conducted in Europe) are randomized, controlled, open-label, NI clinical trials to

© The Author(s) 2016

T. Hamasaki et al., *Group-Sequential Clinical Trials with Multiple Co-Objectives*, JSS Research Series in Statistics, DOI 10.1007/978-4-431-55900-9_6

evaluate the efficacy and safety of peginesatide as the maintenance treatment of anemia in patients with chronic renal failure who were receiving hemodialysis and previously treated with epoetin (Fishbane et al. 2013). Both trials included a 6-week screening period, a 28-week initial dose adjustment period, an 8-week evaluation period, and a longer-term follow-up period (≥ 16 additional weeks). Eligible participants were randomly assigned, in a 2:1 ratio, to receive peginesatide once every 4 weeks or to continue to receive epoetin (epoetin alfa in the EMERALD 1 and epoetin beta in the EMERALD 2) one to three times a week. The frequency and route of administration of epoetin were determined based on the treatment regimen during the screening period. The primary efficacy endpoint was the change from the baseline hemoglobin level during the evaluation period. NI for both trials would be established if the lower limit of the two-sided 95 % confidence interval was -1.0 g per deciliter or higher, indicating that inferiority of greater than -1.0 could be ruled out with reasonable confidence, compared to epoetin.

For NI clinical trials to be valid, two assumptions (constancy and assay sensitivity) must be satisfied (International Conference on Harmonisation of Technical Requirements for Registration of Pharmaceuticals for Human Use (ICH) 2000; D'Agostino et al. 2003; Food and Drug Administration (FDA) 2010; Evans and Follmann 2015). An active intervention which has been shown to be efficacious (e.g., superior to placebo) in a historical trial may be considered as the active control in a NI trial, but the most effective should be selected. The constancy assumption states that the demonstrated effect of the active control over placebo in the historical trial has not changed over time, i.e., would be the same as the effect in the current trial if a placebo group was included. This may not be the case if there were differences in trial conduct (e.g., differences in treatment administration, endpoints, or population) between the historical and current trials. This assumption is not testable in a trial without a concurrent placebo group.

Another important design assumption is assay sensitivity, i.e., the ability for the trial to be able to detect differences between strategies if they truly exist. Otherwise, NI may be concluded simply due to insensitivity of the trial to detect differences. In NI trials, assay sensitivity (essentially making strategies appear similar) can be reduced (intentionally or unintentionally) by diluting effects though subtle choices about design and conduct. Many factors can affect assay sensitivity including poor disease diagnosis, endpoint selection and timing, poor adherence, loss to follow-up, prior therapy, inclusion of subgroups where treatment effects may be small, and use of concomitant therapies. Furthermore, the active control nature of the most NI trials can make clinicians and participants more likely to rate positive outcomes, driving the results toward NI.

The methodologies for two-arm (a test intervention and an effective active control) NI clinical trials have been well established. However, two-arm NI trials often lack the necessary support for the assay sensitivity and constancy assumptions. As a result, inclusion of a third arm (placebo) into the trial has been proposed to address these concerns (Pigeot et al. 2003; Koch and Röhmel 2004; Hauschke and Pigeot 2005a). Regulatory authorities often recommend a use of such a three-arm (test intervention, active control, and placebo) NI trial design (ICH 2000; Committee for Medicinal Products for Human Use (CHMP) 2005; FDA 2010). The three-arm NI trial offers several scientific advantages (ICH 2000). Particularly, these designs provide the opportunity of establishing the validity of the assay sensitivity via a comparison of the placebo with the active control intervention within the trial. Although the three-arm NI design provides such scientific advantages, it also provides challenges: (1) there may be ethical constraints to using a placebo and (2) there is the added complexity of evaluating two distinct objectives: evaluation of (i) the superiority of the active control intervention to placebo (assay sensitivity: AS) and (ii) the NI of the test intervention to the active control intervention. This may result in a trial with too large and impractical of a sample size to conduct. One approach to address this concern is the use of group-sequential designs. The group-sequential design offers the possibility to stop a trial early when evidence is overwhelming and thus offers efficiency (i.e., potentially fewer trial participants and minimizing the amount of time that participants receive a placebo, compared to fixed-sample designs).

In this chapter, we discuss group-sequential designs for three-arm NI clinical trials. We extend two existing approaches for evaluating AS and NI into a group-sequential setting. One approach is discussed by Koch and Röhmel (2004), and Hida and Tango (2011a, 2013) (hereafter we call this "fixed margin approach"), and the other is so-called fraction approach proposed by Pigeot et al. (2003). We consider a three-arm NI trial that has two co-primary objectives: (i) to evaluate whether the control intervention is superior to placebo (AS) and (ii) to evaluate whether the test intervention is not less effective than the control intervention by a prespecified NI margin (NI). Objective (ii) is relevant when the test intervention has advantages over the control (e.g., safer, more convenience, or less costly). On the other hand, in many NI clinical trials, especially in a regulatory setting, demonstrating the superiority of the test intervention to placebo is desirable. However, as Gao and Ware (2008) discuss, if the AS assumption does not hold, then there will be uncertainty regarding whether a NI result means that they are similarly effective or similarly ineffective. In this chapter, when there is a concern about the AS, to make the evaluation of objective (ii) more interpretable, we evaluate a direct comparison of the control intervention with the placebo. For related discussions, please see Hauschke and Pigeot (2005a, b) and Stucke and Kieser (2012).

Three-arm NI clinical trials in a group-sequential setting have been discussed (Li and Gao 2010; Schlömer and Brannath 2013), but methodologies are still needed. Extensions of the fraction approach are discussed by Li and Gao (2010) and the fixed margin approach by Schlömer and Brannath (2013), in a setting of two-stage group-sequential three-arm NI clinical trials with continuous or binary outcomes. We discuss two decision-making frameworks for the two approaches when the primary endpoint is continuous.

6.2 Evaluating Assay Sensitivity and Non-inferiority

6.2.1 Notation and Statistical Setting

Consider a three-arm NI group-sequential clinical trial with a maximum of L planned analyses ($L \geq 2$). Let n_{Tl}, n_{Cl} and n_{Pl} be the cumulative numbers of participants on the test intervention (T), active control intervention (C), and placebo (P) groups, respectively, at the lth interim analysis ($l = 1, \ldots, L$). Let the allocation ratios of the C and the P relative to the T be $n_{Tl} : n_{Cl} : n_{Pl} = 1 : r_C : r_P$, where $r_C(>0)$ and $r_P(>0)$. When the groups are equally sized, $r_C = r_P = 1$. Hence, up to n_{TL}, $n_{CL} = r_C n_{TL}$ and $n_{PL} = r_P n_{TL}$, participants are recruited and randomly assigned to the intervention groups. The sample size required for the final analysis N_L is $N_L = n_{TL} + n_{CL} + n_{PL} = (1 + r_C + r_P)n_{TL}$.

Assume that the group outcomes Y_{Ti}, Y_{Cj}, and Y_{Pm} are independently distributed with means $E[Y_{Ti}] = \mu_T$, $E[Y_{Cj}] = \mu_C$, and $E[Y_{Pm}] = \mu_P$, and common variance $\text{var}[Y_{Ti}] = \text{var}[Y_{Cj}] = \text{var}[Y_{Pm}] = \sigma^2$, respectively ($i = 1, \ldots, n_{TL}$; $j = 1, \ldots, n_{CL}$; $m = 1, \ldots, n_{PL}$), where a larger mean represents a more preferable outcome. For simplicity, the variance σ^2 is assumed to be known.

6.2.2 The Fixed Margin Approach

For the fixed margin approach, the hypotheses for evaluating AS and NI, respectively, are as follows:

$$H_0^{AS}:\mu_C - \mu_P \leq \omega \quad \text{versus} \quad H_1^{AS}:\mu_C - \mu_P > \omega, \tag{6.1}$$

$$H_0^{NI}:\mu_T - \mu_C \leq -\omega \quad \text{versus} \quad H_1^{NI}:\mu_T - \mu_C > -\omega, \tag{6.2}$$

where $\omega(>0)$ is a prespecified NI margin (Hida and Tango 2011a). This approach imposes an extra condition on the hypothesis testing for the AS, that is, superiority of the C to the P is demonstrated with a NI margin ω. However, the key feature of the approach is that the inequalities $\mu_P < \mu_C - \omega < \mu_T$ hold for any value of ω if both of the null hypotheses H_0^{NI} and H_0^{AS} are rejected at the significance level of α for a one-sided test. This means that the superiority of the T relative to the P can be indirectly demonstrated if H_0^{NI} and H_0^{AS} are rejected, without direct comparison of the T with the P. This avoids introduction of further complexities in adjustment to the Type I or Type II errors (Hida and Tango 2011a).

We are now interested in hypothesis testing for AS and NI based on the fixed margin approach within a group-sequential setting. The corresponding statistics for testing hypotheses (6.1) and (6.2) at the lth interim analysis are given by

$$Z_l^{AS} = \frac{\bar{Y}_{Cl} - \bar{Y}_{Pl} - \omega}{\sigma\sqrt{1/n_{Cl} + 1/n_{Pl}}} \quad \text{and} \quad Z_l^{NI} = \frac{\bar{Y}_{Tl} - \bar{Y}_{Cl} + \omega}{\sigma\sqrt{1/n_{Tl} + 1/n_{Cl}}}$$

where $\bar{Y}_{Tl}$, $\bar{Y}_{Cl}$, and $\bar{Y}_{Pl}$ are the sample means in the T, the C, and the P, respectively, at the lth interim analysis, given by $\bar{Y}_{Tl} = \left(\sum_{i=1}^{n_{Tl}} Y_{Ti}\right)/n_{Tl}$, $\bar{Y}_{Cl} = \left(\sum_{j=1}^{n_{Cl}} Y_{Cj}\right)/n_{Cl}$, and $\bar{Y}_{Pl} = \left(\sum_{m=1}^{n_{Pl}} Y_{Pm}\right)/n_{Pl}$. Then, for large samples, (Z_l^{AS}, Z_l^{NI}) is approximately bivariate normally distributed with the correlation

$$\text{corr}\left[Z_l^{AS}, Z_l^{NI}\right] = -\sqrt{\frac{n_{Tl}n_{Pl}}{(n_{Tl} + n_{Cl})(n_{Cl} + n_{Pl})}} = -\sqrt{\frac{r_P}{(1 + r_C)(r_C + r_P)}} = \rho.$$

The correlation is determined by the allocation ratios r_C and r_P (Hida and Tango 2011a). The two statistics (Z_l^{AS}, Z_l^{NI}) are always negatively correlated and become closer to zero as r_C and r_P are larger. The correlation is $\rho = -0.5$ if the intervention groups are equally sized, i.e., $r_C = r_P = 1$. Furthermore, the joint distribution of $(Z_1^{AS}, Z_1^{NI}, \ldots, Z_l^{AS}, Z_l^{NI}, \ldots, Z_L^{AS}, Z_L^{NI})$ is $2L$ multivariate normally distributed with correlations given by $\text{corr}\left[Z_{l'}^{AS}, Z_l^{AS}\right] = \text{corr}\left[Z_{l'}^{NI}, Z_l^{NI}\right] = \sqrt{n_{Tl'}/n_{Tl}}$, and $\text{corr}[Z_{l'}^{AS}, Z_l^{NI}] = \text{corr}[Z_{l'}^{NI}, Z_l^{AS}] = \rho\sqrt{n_{Tl'}/n_{Tl}}$ $(1 \leq l' \leq l \leq L)$ since Z_l^{AS} and Z_l^{NI} can be rewritten as

$$Z_l^{AS} = \frac{\sqrt{n_{Tl}}(\bar{Y}_{Cl} - \bar{Y}_{Pl} - \omega)}{\sigma\sqrt{1/r_C + 1/r_P}} \quad \text{and} \quad Z_l^{NI} = \frac{\sqrt{n_{Tl}}(\bar{Y}_{Tl} - \bar{Y}_{Cl} + \omega)}{\sigma\sqrt{1 + 1/r_C}}.$$

6.2.3   The Fraction Approach

For the fraction approach, the hypotheses for evaluating AS and NI, respectively, are as follows:

$$H_0^{AS} : \mu_C - \mu_P \leq 0 \quad \text{versus} \quad H_1^{AS} : \mu_C - \mu_P > 0, \tag{6.3}$$

$$H_0^{NI} : (\mu_T - \mu_P)/(\mu_C - \mu_P) \leq \theta \quad \text{versus} \quad H_1^{NI} : (\mu_T - \mu_P)/(\mu_C - \mu_P) > \theta, \tag{6.4}$$

where θ $(0 < \theta < 1)$ is prespecified and determined by $\theta = 1 - \omega/(\mu_C - \mu_P)$ as a fraction of the difference between μ_C and μ_P, using the NI margin ω (Pigeot et al. 2003). In addition, hypothesis testing is logically ordered, i.e., H_0^{AS} is tested first, and then H_0^{NI} is tested if and only if H_0^{AS} is rejected at the prespecified significance level of α. If both null hypotheses H_0^{AS} and H_0^{NI} are rejected, then $\mu_T > \mu_P$ irrespective of θ since $\mu_T - \mu_P > \theta(\mu_C - \mu_P) > 0$. Many authors have discussed the fraction approach in fixed-sample designs; binary outcomes are discussed by Tang and Tang (2004) and Kieser and Friede (2007), time-to-event outcomes by Mielke et al. (2008) and Kombrink et al. (2013), and continuous outcomes with heterogeneous variances by Hasler et al. (2008).

We focus on hypothesis testing based on the fraction approach within a group-sequential setting. Assuming $\mu_C - \mu_P > 0$, the hypotheses (6.4) can be rewritten as

$$H_0^{NI}: \mu_T - \theta\mu_C - (1 - \theta)\mu_P \leq 0 \quad \text{versus} \quad H_1^{NI}: \mu_T - \theta\mu_C - (1 - \theta)\mu_P > 0.$$

The corresponding statistics for testing hypotheses (6.3) and (6.4) at the lth interim analysis are given by

$$Z_l^{AS} = \frac{\bar{Y}_{Cl} - \bar{Y}_{Pl}}{\sigma\sqrt{1/n_{Cl} + 1/n_{Pl}}} \quad \text{and} \quad Z_l^{NI} = \frac{\bar{Y}_{Tl} - \theta\bar{Y}_{Cl} - (1 - \theta)\bar{Y}_{Pl}}{\sigma\sqrt{1/n_{Tl} + \theta^2/n_{Cl} + (1 - \theta)^2/n_{Pl}}}.$$

For large sample, (Z_l^{AS}, Z_l^{NI}) is approximately bivariate normally distributed and the joint distribution of $(Z_1^{AS}, Z_1^{NI} \ldots, Z_l^{AS}, Z_l^{NI}, \ldots, Z_L^{AS}, Z_L^{NI})$ is $2L$ multivariate normally distributed with their correlations given by the same correlation structure as the fixed margin approach. The correlations of Z_l^{AS} and Z_l^{NI} are given by

$$\text{corr}\left[Z_l^{AS}, Z_l^{NI}\right] = \frac{-\theta/r_C + (1 - \theta)/r_P}{\sqrt{1 + \theta^2/r_C + (1 - \theta)^2/r_P}\sqrt{1/r_C + 1/r_P}} = \rho.$$

The correlation is determined by the fraction θ and the allocation ratios r_C and r_P. When the intervention groups are equally sized, i.e., $r_C = r_P = 1$, it is $\rho = (1 - 2\theta)/2\sqrt{1 - \theta + \theta^2}$, and $\rho = 0$ if $\theta = 0.5$.

There are important differences in the two approaches (Röhmel and Pigeot 2011; Hida and Tango 2011a, b; Stucke and Kieser 2012). Specifically, the concept of "assay sensitivity" is different. A different conclusion is driven from the two approaches when $\mu_C - \omega < \mu_P < \mu_C$ is true (Hida and Tango 2011b). The fraction approach can reject H_0^{NI}, but the fixed margin approach cannot. Whether the fraction approach can allow demonstration of NI of the T to the C is questionable under $\mu_C - \omega < \mu_P$. For further discussion, please see Röhmel and Pigeot (2011), Hida and Tango (2011b), and Stucke and Kieser (2012).

6.3 Decision-Making Frameworks and Stopping Rules

We consider two decision-making frameworks associated with hypothesis testing. The first decision-making framework is flexible, where testing hypotheses for AS and NI are logically ordered similarly as in the fraction approach, i.e., NI is evaluated only after the AS is demonstrated and a trial is terminated if H_0^{AS} and H_0^{NI} are rejected at any interim analysis (i.e., not necessarily simultaneously) (DF-A). The other framework is relatively simple and a special case of DF-A, where a clinical trial is terminated if and only if both H_0^{AS} and H_0^{NI} are rejected simultaneously at the same interim analysis (DF-B). We describe the two decision-making frameworks, corresponding stopping rules and power definitions.

DF-A: Under DF-A, a trial stops if the AS and the NI are achieved at any interim analysis (i.e., not necessarily simultaneously). NI is evaluated only after the AS is demonstrated. If AS is demonstrated but NI is not, then the trial continues and subsequent hypothesis testing is repeatedly conducted only for NI until the NI is demonstrated. The stopping rule based on DF-A is formally given as follows:

At the lth interim analysis ($l = l', \ldots, L - 1$),

if $Z_{l'}^{AS} > Z_{l'}^{AS}$ for some $l'(1 \leq l' \leq l)$ and $Z_l^{NI} > c_l^{NI}$, then reject H_0^{NI} and stop the trial
otherwise, continue the trial,

at the Lth analysis,

if $Z_{l'}^{AS} > c_{l'}^{AS}$ for some l' and $Z_L^{NI} > c_L^{NI}$, then reject H_0^{NI},
otherwise, do not reject H_0^{NI}.

where c_l^{AS} and c_l^{NI} are the critical boundaries at the lth interim analysis, which are constant and selected separately for AS and NI to preserve the Type I error of α for each hypothesis, using any group-sequential method such as Lan–DeMets error-spending method (Lan and DeMets 1983), analogously to a trial with a single primary objective. For example, consider a three-arm NI clinical trial with a maximum number of planned analyses $L = 4$ and equally spaced increments of information, and the O'Brien–Fleming-type boundary (OF) (O'Brien and Fleming 1979) is used to reject the null hypothesis for the AS and NI tests with the same significance level of $\alpha = 2.5\%$ for a one-sided test. The boundaries for each analysis are 4.3326, 2.9631, 2.3590, and 2.0141, respectively. If the AS test is statistically significant at the third analysis, then the NI test is evaluated twice with the critical boundary of 2.3590 at the third analysis and 2.0141 at the final analysis as if the significance level for the NI test has been already spent at the first and second analyses despite no test being conducted. Even if the AS test is statistically significant at the third analysis, the remaining significance level of 1.5 % (=2.5 − 1.0) is not reallocated to the hypothesis test for NI. If the remaining significance level of 1.5 % for the AS test is reallocated to the hypothesis test for NI, then the size of the hypothesis tests for AS and NI is at most $\alpha = 4.0\%$ (=1.5 + 2.5) since the test is the intersection–union.

Therefore, the overall power for rejecting the both H_0^{AS} and H_0^{NI} under H_1^{AS} and H_1^{NI} in DF-A is

$$1 - \beta = \Pr\left[\bigcup_{1 \le l' \le l \le L} \left\{\left\{Z_{l'}^{AS} > c_{l'}^{AS}\right\} \cap \left\{Z_l^{NI} > c_l^{NI}\right\}\right\} \Big| H_1^{AS} \cap H_1^{NI}\right]. \quad (6.5)$$

This power (6.5) can be evaluated using the numerical integration method in Genz (1992) or using other methods.

When using the fixed margin approach, DF-A allows for dropping of the P if AS is demonstrated at the interim. However, when using the fraction approach, DF-A cannot allow this as the test statistics for the NI includes the amount of $\bar{Y}_{Pl}$.

DF-B: Under DF-B, a trial is stopped if AS and NI are demonstrated at the same interim analysis simultaneously. Otherwise, the trial will continue and the subsequent hypothesis testing is repeatedly conducted for both AS and NI until simultaneous significance is reached. The stopping rule based on DF-B is formally given as follows:

At the lth interim analysis ($l = 1, \ldots, L - 1$),

if $Z_l^{AS} > c_l^{AS}$ and $Z_l^{NI} > c_l^{NI}$ simultaneously, then reject H_0^{AS} and H_0^{NI}, and stop the trial,
otherwise, continue the trial,

at the Lth analysis

if $Z_L^{AS} > c_L^{AS}$ and $Z_L^{NI} > c_L^{NI}$, then reject H_0^{AS} and H_0^{NI},
otherwise, do not reject H_0^{AS} and H_0^{NI}.

Similarly as in the DF-A, the critical boundaries at the lth interim analysis c_l^{AS} and c_l^{NI} are constant and selected separately for the AS and NI tests to preserve the Type I error of α for each hypothesis, using any group-sequential method, analogously to a trial with a single primary objective. Therefore, the overall power for rejecting both H_0^{AS} and H_0^{NI} under H_1^{AS} and H_1^{NI} in DF-B is

$$1 - \beta = \Pr\left[\bigcup_{l=1}^{L} \left\{\left\{Z_l^{NI} > c_l^{NI}\right\} \cap \left\{Z_l^{AS} > c_l^{AS}\right\}\right\} \Big| H_1^{AS} \cap H_1^{NI}\right]. \quad (6.6)$$

This power (6.6) can also be numerically assessed by using multivariate normal integrals.

Based on the powers for DF-A (6.5) and DF-B (6.6) discussed above, in a group-sequential setting, similarly we describe two sample size concepts, the maximum sample size (MSS) and the average sample number (ASN) as in Chap. 2.

The MSS is the sample size required for the final analysis to achieve the desired overall power $1 - \beta$ for rejecting both null hypotheses for AS and NI. The MSS is the smallest integer not less than N_L satisfying the desired power for a group-sequential strategy at the prespecified hypothetical values of parameters μ_T, μ_C, and μ_P, σ^2, and ω (or θ) with Fisher's information time for the interim analyses. The ASN is the expected sample size under hypothetical reference values and provides information regarding the number of participants anticipated in a group-sequential clinical trial in order to reach a decision point. The definitions of ASNs corresponding to the two decision-making frameworks for the fixed margin and fraction approaches are given in the Appendix D.

To identify the value of n_{TL} or N_L, a simple strategy is to implement a grid search to gradually increase (or decrease) n_{TL} until the power under n_{TL} exceeds (or falls below) the desired power. The grid search often requires considerable computing time, especially with a larger number of planned analyses, or a small standardized mean difference. As mentioned in Chap. 2, to reduce the computing time, the Newton–Raphson algorithm in Sugimoto et al. (2012) or the basic linear interpolation algorithm in Hamasaki et al. (2013) may be utilized.

6.4 Illustration

We illustrate the concepts with an example from the Rotigotine trial (Mizuno et al. 2014). The study was designed to evaluate the superiority of transdermal rotigotine to placebo, and NI to ropinirole, in Japanese Parkinson's disease patients on concomitant levodopa therapy. The primary variable was the change in the unified Parkinson's disease rating scale (UPDRS) Part III (ON state) sum score from baseline to week 16 of the treatment period [end of treatment (EOT)]. For the sample size calculation for the trial, the change from baseline in UPDRS was assumed to be 5.4 for the rotigotine, 5.0 for the ropinirole, and zero for placebo with a common standard deviation of 9.0 among the groups. In addition, the NI margin of rotigotine to ropinirole was 2.5. Based on these assumptions, the MSS and ASN are calculated for evaluating AS and NI with 80 % power at the 2.5 % significance level for a one-sided test, when using the fixed margin and fraction approaches based on DF-A and DF-B with the number of planned analyses $L = 2, 3$, and 4. The three allocation ratios $n_{Tl} : n_{Cl} : n_{Pl}$ considered are (i) 1:1:1 ($r_C = r_P = 1$), (ii) 2:2:1 ($r_C = 1, r_P = 1/2$), and (iii) 2:1:1 ($r_C = r_P = 1/2$). The critical boundaries are determined by using the Lan–DeMets error-spending method with equally spaced increments of information. The four critical boundary combinations considered are as follows: OF for both AS and NI (OF-OF), Pocock-type boundary (PC) (Pocock 1977) for both AS and NI (PC-PC), OF for AS and PC for NI (OF-PC), and PC for AS and OF for NI (PC-OF). Furthermore, for the fixed margin approach based on DF-A, the ASN is calculated under H_1^{AS} and H_1^{NI} in two ways: In one strategy, the placebo group is not discontinued until NI is demonstrated even when AS is

Table 6.1 The MSS and ASN for demonstrating the AS and NI based on the fixed margin approach with 80 % power at the 2.5 % significance level for a one-sided test, where the mean changes from baseline in UPDRS are $\mu_T = 5.4$, $\mu_C = 5.0$, and $\mu_P = 0.0$ with a common standard deviation of $\sigma = 9.0$

Decision-making framework	L	Critical boundary combination	$r_C = r_P = 1$			$r_C = 1, r_P = 1/2$			$r_C = r_P = 1/2$		
			MSS	ASN1	ASN2	MSS	ASN1	ASN2	MSS	ASN1	ASN2
Fixed sample	1		717			800			874		
DF-A	2	OF-OF	720	713	694	803	786	776	878	870	853
		PC-PC	801	681	655	893	733	722	976	821	801
		OF-PC	759	726	713	820	778	772	906	870	860
		PC-OF	771	730	681	880	797	772	956	893	851
	3	OF-OF	726	668	650	810	728	721	886	809	795
		PC-PC	834	674	641	930	724	709	1016	812	786
		OF-PC	774	688	675	833	734	728	920	819	809
		PC-OF	795	690	644	915	763	738	990	842	805
	4	OF-OF	732	652	632	815	711	702	890	788	773
		PC-PC	852	668	633	950	717	700	1038	804	777
		OF-PC	786	677	662	843	719	713	930	803	792
		PC-OF	810	681	634	933	748	724	1010	831	793
DF-B	2	OF-OF	720	713	–	803	786	–	878	870	–
		PC-PC	810	686	–	900	737	–	986	826	–
		OF-PC	759	726	–	820	778	–	906	870	–
		PC-OF	789	743	–	900	810	–	980	909	–
	3	OF-OF	729	670	–	810	729	–	886	809	–
		PC-PC	846	684	–	943	733	–	1030	824	–
		OF-PC	774	688	–	835	735	–	922	820	–
		PC-OF	813	707	–	935	782	–	1014	865	–
	4	OF-OF	735	654	–	815	711	–	894	791	–
		PC-PC	864	680	–	963	729	–	1054	820	–
		OF-PC	786	677	–	843	719	–	932	805	–
		PC-OF	828	698	–	955	769	–	1034	854	–

The prespecified NI margin is $\omega = 2.5$. The three allocation ratios $n_{TI} : n_{CI} : n_{PI}$ considered are (i) 1:1:1 ($r_C = r_P = 1$), (ii) 2:2:1 ($r_C = 1, r_P = 1/2$), and (iii) 2:1:1 ($r_C = r_P = 1/2$). The critical boundaries are determined by using the Lan–DeMets error-spending method with equally spaced increments of information. The four critical boundary combinations considered are O'Brien–Fleming-type boundary (OF) for both AS and NI (OF-OF), Pocock-type boundary (PC) for both AS and NI (PC-PC), OF for AS and PC for NI (OF-PC), and PC for AS and OF for NI (PC-OF)

Table 6.2 The MSS and ASN for demonstrating the AS and NI based on the fraction approach with 80 % power at the 2.5 % significance level for a one-sided test, where the mean changes from baseline in UPDRS are $\mu_T = 5.4$, $\mu_C = 5.0$, and $\mu_P = 0.0$ with a common standard deviation of $\sigma = 9.0$

Decision-making framework	L	Critical boundary combination	$r_C = r_P = 1$			$r_C = 1, r_P = 1/2$			$r_C = r_P = 1/2$		
			MSS	ASN1	ASN2	MSS	ASN1	ASN2	MSS	ASN1	ASN2
Fixed sample	1		351			353			338		
DF-A	2	OF-OF	351	336	–	353	337	–	340	329	–
		PC-PC	393	312	–	395	315	–	380	310	–
		OF-PC	396	339	–	395	343	–	376	338	–
		PC-OF	354	330	–	360	333	–	352	328	–
	3	OF-OF	354	312	–	358	315	–	344	308	–
		PC-PC	411	306	–	413	308	–	396	304	–
		OF-PC	414	335	–	410	335	–	388	326	–
		PC-OF	360	312	–	368	317	–	358	311	–
	4	OF-OF	357	304	–	360	307	–	346	300	–
		PC-PC	420	304	–	423	305	–	406	302	–
		OF-PC	420	326	–	418	328	–	396	320	–
		PC-OF	363	304	–	370	308	–	362	304	–
DF-B	2	OF-OF	351	336	–	353	337	–	340	329	–
		PC-PC	393	312	–	395	315	–	382	311	–
		OF-PC	396	339	–	395	343	–	376	338	–
		PC-OF	357	332	–	363	335	–	354	330	–
	3	OF-OF	354	312	–	358	315	–	344	308	–
		PC-PC	411	307	–	413	309	–	398	306	–
		OF-PC	414	335	–	410	335	–	388	326	–
		PC-OF	363	314	–	370	319	–	362	315	–
	4	OF-OF	357	304	–	360	307	–	346	300	–
		PC-PC	420	304	–	423	306	–	408	304	–
		OF-PC	420	326	–	418	328	–	396	320	–
		PC-OF	366	306	–	375	312	–	368	309	–

The prespecified NI margin is $\theta = 0.5$. The three allocation ratios $n_{T_i} : n_{C_i} : n_{P_i}$ considered are (i) 1:1:1 ($r_C = r_P = 1$), (ii) 2:2:1 ($r_C = 1, r_P = 1/2$), and (iii) 2:1:1 ($r_C = r_P = 1/2$). The critical boundaries are determined by using the Lan–DeMets error-spending method with equally spaced increments of information. The four critical boundary combinations considered are OF for both AS and NI (OF-OF), PC for both AS and NI (PC-PC), OF for AS and PC for NI (OF-PC), and PC for AS and OF for NI (PC-OF)

demonstrated at an interim analysis (ASN1), while in the other strategy the P is discontinued when AS is demonstrated at an interim analysis (ASN2). The definitions of ASN1 and ASN2 are given in Appendix D. Tables 6.1 and 6.2 summarize the calculated sample sizes.

For both the fixed margin and fraction approaches, in all of the critical boundary combinations and allocation ratios, there is a modest difference in the MSS and ASN between the DF-A and DF-B although DF-A provides a slightly smaller sample size than DF-B.

For the fixed margin approach, the smallest MSS is given by OF-OF and the largest by PC-PC in all of the allocation ratios. The smallest ASN1 is associated with OF-OF or PC-PC and the largest with PC-OF. The largest ASN2 is provided by PC-OF or OF-PC in all of the allocation ratios. If three interims and one final analysis are planned (i.e., $L = 4$) based on DF-A, then the total MSS is 732 for OF-OF, 852 for PC-PC, and 786 for OF-PC, and 810 for PC-OF. The total ASN1 is 652 for OF-OF, 668 for PC-PC, 677 for OF-PC, and 681 for PC-OF, and the total ASN2 is 632 for OF-OF, 633 for PC-PC, 662 for OF-PC, and 634 for PC-OF. With DF-B, then the total MSS is 735 for OF-OF, 864 for PC-PC and 786 for OF-PC, and 828 for PC-OF. The total ASN1 is 654 for OF-OF, 680 for PC-PC, 677 for OF-PC, and 698 for PC-OF.

For the fraction approach, the smallest MSS is provided by OF-OF and the largest by OF-PC or PC-PC in all of the allocation ratios. The smallest ASN1 is consistently produced with PC-PC and the largest with OF-PC. When the number of participants is equally sized among the groups, without any interim analysis, the total fixed-sample size is 351. If three interims and one final analysis are planned based on DF-A, then the total MSS is 357 for OF-OF, 420 for PC-PC and 420 for OF-PC, and 363 for PC-OF. The total ASN1 is 304 for OF-OF, 304 for PC-PC, 326 for OF-PC, and 304 for PC-OF.

6.5   Summary

NI clinical trials recently have received a great deal of attention by regulatory authorities (CHMP 2005; FDA 2010) and in the clinical trials' literature [e.g., extensive reference found in Rothmann et al. (2011)]. NI clinical trials have complexities requiring careful design, monitoring, analyses, and reporting. When designing NI clinical trials, the constancy and AS are the important assumptions. The selection of the active control for a NI trial should be done carefully, ensuring that it has demonstrated and precisely measured superiority over placebo and that its effect has not changed compared to the historical trials that demonstrated its efficacy (constancy assumption). To assess these issues in regulatory medical product development, the use of three-arm NI design that includes a test intervention, an active control intervention, and a placebo has been considered as a gold standard design, although this design may not be possible due to ethical constraints and the impracticalities of large sample sizes required for three-arm trials.

In this chapter, we discuss three-arm NI clinical trials and extend two existing approaches, i.e., the fixed margin and fraction approaches, for evaluating AS and NI to a group-sequential setting with two decision-making frameworks.

With the result discussed in Ochiai et al. (2016), the findings are summarized as follows:

- The decision-making frameworks of DF-A and DF-B for the fixed margin and the fraction approaches provide the possibility of stopping a trial early when evidence is overwhelming, thus offering efficiency (e.g., an ASN potentially 4–15 % fewer than the fixed-sample designs with equally sized groups and four analyses).
- There are no major differences in both MSS and ASN between DF-A and DF-B for the fixed margin and the fraction approaches, although DF-A is slightly more powerful than DF-B. By using the DF-A for the fixed margin approach, the time that participants are exposed to placebo can be minimized as the DF-A allows dropping of the placebo group if AS has been demonstrated at an interim analysis.
- For the fixed margin approach, selecting the OF-type boundary for both AS and NI could lead to fewer participants for the MSS and the ASN compared with other critical boundary combinations. On the other hand, for the fraction approach, selecting the OF-type boundary for both AS and NI, or the PC-type boundary for AS and the OF-type boundary for NI provides better efficiency with respect to the MSS and the ASN compared with other critical boundary combinations.

We caution that these findings are based on one set of design parameter configurations except for the allocation ratio. Further investigation is required to evaluate how the power and Type I error rate behave under other design assumptions.

References

Committee for Medicinal Products for Human Use (CHMP) (2005) Guideline on the choice of the non-inferiority margin. Available at: http://www.ema.europa.eu/docs/en_GB/document_library/Scientific_guideline/2009/09/WC500003636.pdf. Accessed 25 Nov 2015

D'Agostino RB, Massaro JM, Sullivan LM (2003) Non-inferiority trials: design concepts and issues—the encounters of academic consultants in statistics. Stat Med 22:169–186

Evans SR, Follmann D (2015) Fundamentals and innovation in antibiotic trials. Stat Biopharm Res 7:331–336

Fishbane S, Schiller B, Locatelli F, Covic AC, Provenzano R, Wiecek A, Levin NW, Kaplan M, Macdougall IC, Francisco C, Mayo MR, Polu KR, Duliege AM, Besarab A, for the EMERALD Study Groups (2013) Peginesatide in patients with anemia undergoing hemodialysis. New Engl J Med 368:307–319

Food and Drug Administration (FDA) (2010) Guidance for industry non-inferiority trials. U.S. Department of health and human services food and drug administration. Rockville, MD, USA.

Available at: http://www.fda.gov/downloads/Drugs/GuidanceComplianceRegulatoryInformation/Guidances/UCM202140.pdf. Accessed 25 Nov 2015

Gao P, Ware JH (2008) Assessing non-inferiority: a combination approach. Stat Med 27:392–406

Genz A (1992) Numerical computation of multivariate normal probabilities. J Comput Graph Stat 1:141–149

Hauschke D, Pigeot I (2005a) Establishing efficacy of a new experimental treatment in the 'gold standard' design. Biometrical J 47:782–786

Hauschke D, Pigeot I (2005b) Rejoinder to "establishing efficacy of a new experimental treatment in the 'gold standard' design". Biometrical J 47:797–798

Hasler M, Vonk R, Hothorn LA (2008) Assessing non-inferiority of a new treatment in a three-arm trial in the presence of heteroscedasticity. Stat Med 27:490–503

Hamasaki T, Sugimoto T, Evans SR, Sozu T (2013) Sample size determination for clinical trials with co-primary outcomes: exponential event times. Pharm Stat 12:28–34

Hida E, Tango T (2011a) On the three-arm non-inferiority trial including a placebo with a prespecified margin. Stat Med 30:224–231

Hida E, Tango T (2011b) Response to Joachim Röhmel and Iris Pigeot. Stat Med 30:3165

Hida E, Tango T (2013) Three-arm noninferiority trials with a prespecified margin for inference of the difference in the proportions of binary endpoints. J Biopharm Stat 23:774–789

International Conference on Harmonisation of Technical Requirements for Registration of Pharmaceuticals for Human Use (ICH) (2000) ICH harmonised tripartite guideline E10: Choice of control group and related issues in clinical trials. July 2000. Available at: http://www.ich.org/fileadmin/Public_Web_Site/ICH_Products/Guidelines/Efficacy/E10/Step4/E10_Guideline.pdf. Accessed 25 Nov 2015

Kieser M, Friede T (2007) Planning and analysis of three-arm non-inferiority trials with binary endpoints. Stat Med 26:253–273

Koch A, Röhmel J (2004) Hypothesis testing in the 'gold standard' design for proving the efficacy of an experimental treatment. J Biopharm Stat 14:315–325

Kombrink K, Munk A, Friede T (2013) Design and semiparametric analysis of non-inferiority trials with active and placebo control for censored time-to-event data. Stat Med 32:3055–3066

Lan KKG, DeMets DL (1983) Discrete sequential boundaries for clinical trials. Biometrika 70:659–663

Li G, Gao S (2010) A group sequential type design for three-arm non-inferiority trials with binary endpoints. Biometrical J 52:504–518

Mielke M, Munk A, Schacht A (2008) The assessment of non-inferiority in a gold standard design with censored, exponentially distributed endpoints. Stat Med 27:5093–5110

Mizuno Y, Nomoto M, Hasegawa K, Hattori N, Kondo T, Murata M, Takeuchi M, Takahashi M, Tomida T, on behalf of the Rotigotine Trial Group (2014) Rotigotine vs ropinirole in advanced stage Parkinson's disease: a double-blind study. Parkinsonism and Related Disorders 20:1388–1393

O'Brien PC, Fleming TR (1979) A multiple testing procedure for clinical trials. Biometrics 35:549–556

Ochiai T, Hamasaki T, Evans SR, Asakura K, Ohno Y (2016) Group-sequential three-arm noninferiority clinical trial designs. J Biopharm Stat (First published online: 18 Feb 2016 as doi:10.1080/10543406.2016.1148710)

Pigeot I, Schäfer J, Röhmel J, Hauschke D (2003) Assessing non-inferiority of a new treatment in a three-arm clinical trial including a placebo. Stat Med 22:883–899

Pocock SJ (1977) Group sequential methods in the design and analysis of clinical trials. Biometrika 64:191–199

Röhmel J, Pigeot I (2011) Statistical strategies for the analysis of clinical trials with an experimental treatment, an active control and placebo, and a prespecified fixed non-inferiority margin for the difference in means. Stat Med 30:3162–3164

Rothmann MD, Wiens BL, Chan ISF (2011) Design and analysis of non-inferiority trials. Chapman and Hall/CRC Press, Boca Raton

Schlömer P, Brannath W (2013) Group sequential designs for three-arm 'gold standard' non-inferiority trials with fixed margin. Stat Med 32:4875–4899

Stucke K, Kieser M (2012) A general approach for sample size calculation for the three-arm 'gold standard' non-inferiority design. Stat Med 31:3579–3596

Sugimoto T, Sozu T, Hamasaki T (2012) A convenient formula for sample size calculations in clinical trials with multiple co-primary continuous endpoints. Pharm Stat 11:118–128

Tang ML, Tang NS (2004) Test of noninferiority via rate difference for three-arm clinical trials with placebo. J Biopharm Stat 14:337–347

Chapter 7
Future Developments

Abstract Chapters 1–6 focus on selected emerging statistical issues in clinical trials. This work provides a foundation for designing randomized trials with other design features. This includes clinical trials with more than two interventions (e.g., dose-selection clinical trials): trials with time-to-event endpoints and trials with targeted subgroups and enrichment clinical trial designs. In Chap. 7, we briefly discuss the issues in the design of these trials.

Keywords Endpoint selection · Enrichment clinical trial designs · Multiple-arm · Subgroup analysis · Time-to-event outcomes

7.1 Introduction

This book discusses group-sequential designs in (i) superiority clinical trials for comparing the effect of two interventions with multiple endpoints, and (ii) three-arm non-inferiority clinical trials for evaluating assay sensitivity and non-inferiority of a test intervention to a control intervention. Our discussion has focused on co-primary endpoints in a group-sequential setting. We have only briefly discussed trials with multiple primary endpoints with a prespecified non-ordering of endpoints. For three-arm non-inferiority clinical trials, we only discuss trials designed with a single endpoint.

However, this work provides a foundation for designing randomized trials with other design features. These include clinical trials with more than two interventions (e.g., dose-selection clinical trials): trials with time-to-event endpoints and trials with targeted subgroups. In Chap. 7, we briefly discuss the issues in the design of such trials.

T. Hamasaki et al., *Group-Sequential Clinical Trials with Multiple Co-Objectives*,
JSS Research Series in Statistics, DOI 10.1007/978-4-431-55900-9_7

7.2   Multiple Intervention Arms

In clinical trials with multiple intervention arms, clarification of the trial objective is paramount. Objectives may include evaluating if *all* interventions are superior (or non-inferior) to a control or if *at least one* intervention is superior (or non-inferior) to a control. For the latter objective, methods for group-sequential and modern adaptive designs for multiple intervention arms have been discussed (e.g., Thall et al. 1989; Follmann et al. 1994; Stallard and Todd 2003, 2008; König et al. 2008; Magirr et al. 2012). Further investigation is needed for group-sequential and adaptive designs in more complex clinical trial settings, e.g., multiple intervention arms with multiple endpoints and targeted subpopulations.

7.3   Multiple Event-Time Outcomes

Methods for time-to-event outcomes are more complex than binary or continuous endpoints. Considerable care is needed to design event-time trials in a group-sequential setting. As discussed in Sugimoto et al. (2013) and Hamasaki et al. (2013) in the fixed-sample designs, the magnitude of the association among the time-to-event outcomes may depend on time. For example, the outcomes may be less correlated in earlier stages but more highly correlated in later stages.

The censoring mechanism further complicates the design of these trials. For example, coinfection/comorbidity trials may utilize primary endpoints to evaluate multiple comorbidities; e.g., a trial evaluating therapies to treat Kaposi's sarcoma (KS) in HIV-infected individuals may have the time to KS progression and the time to HIV virologic failure, as primary endpoints. Both events are non-fatal and neither event-time is censored by the other event. In new anticancer drug trials, the most commonly used primary endpoint is overall survival (OS) defined as the time from randomization until death from any cause. OS often requires long follow-up periods after disease progression leading to long and expensive studies. Therefore, in addition to OS, as a primary endpoint, many trials evaluate the time from randomization to the first of tumor progression (TTP) or progression-free survival (PFS) which is composite of tumor progression and death. In this example, a death event would censor TTP: Death is a competing risk for TTP but not vice versa. This is referred to as "semi-competing risks" (Fine et al. 2001).

Lastly, when extending the methods discussed in Chaps. 2–4 to time-to-event outcomes, as pointed out by Hung et al. (2015), a complex issue is how to allocate the significance level to each interim analysis as the amount of information for the endpoints may vary at a particular interim time-point of the trial.

7.4 Endpoint Selection Designs

Typically, the primary endpoints are the outcomes which provide the most clinically relevant and convincing evidence directly related to the primary objective of a clinical trial (e.g., the variable used to compare the effect difference of two treatment groups) [the International Conference on Harmonisation of Technical Requirements for Registration of Pharmaceuticals for Human Use (ICH) E9 Guideline (1998)]. The primary endpoints should be carefully described in the protocol as it sets the stage for much of the rest of the trial protocol and trial design. For example, the sample size is determined based on the primary endpoint. Failure to prespecify endpoints, especially in conformation clinical trials, can introduce bias into a trial and creates opportunities for manipulation. However, due to the recent technological advances in obtaining a wide variety of measurements from participants in the trial, new information such as identification of better markers or surrogate outcome measures may come to light that could merit changes to endpoints during the course of a trial (Evans 2007). While changes can allow incorporation of up-to-date knowledge into the trial design, such changes to endpoints can also compromise the scientific integrity of a trial.

In early-phase explanatory clinical trials, the primary objective is often to evaluate whether a test intervention is active enough to justify later-phase trials. There may be serval outcomes available to evaluate the multidimensional effects of the intervention. An optimal go/no-go decision relies heavily on how to select outcomes which can characterize the intervention's effect appropriately. One strategy for go/no-go decision-making with endpoint selection is to use an extension of the method using the futility critical boundary discussed in Chap. 4. The decision-making framework is to stop measurement of an endpoint if its test statistic has already crossed the futility critical boundary, but otherwise continue measurement. If all of the statistics for the endpoints under consideration cross the futility critical boundary, then the trial is terminated.

Alternatively, a conditional power (CP) approach related to the methods discussed in Chap. 3 can be considered. A cutoff value is determined based on CP, and measurement is stopped on an endpoint if its CP is lower than the cutoff value, but otherwise measurement continues. Furthermore, an extension to "predicted intervals" to a multiple endpoint setting (Evans et al. 2007; Li et al. 2009) will provide information regarding the potential effect size estimates and associated precision with endpoint measurement continuation, thus providing investigators with a better understanding of the pros and cons associated with continuation of endpoint measurement.

7.5 Enrichment Designs and Subgroup Analyses

Modern genomic studies suggest that many diseases once believed to be homogeneous are heterogeneous. If clinical or pharmacogenomic markers can reliably identify distinct diseases can be developed, then empirical-based medicine can be transformed to "stratified medicine." The markers may be used to select the best therapeutic strategy for individual patients. The important and challenging task is to identify and confirm a subgroup of patients with a positive benefit: risk balance when treated with an intervention (Ondra et al. 2015).

When a disease is heterogeneous or the intervention can target a specific mechanism of action related to disease subtypes, use of conventional clinical trial design may not suffice. Conventional trials generally assume homogeneous treatment effect for all participants in the trial. When markers can precisely identify individuals with a high probability of response to an intervention, clinical trials could focus on such individuals. Conducting a trial in subgroup patients with a potentially high response is termed "enrichment." Referring to Food and Drug Administration (FDA) guidance on "Enrichment Strategies for Clinical Trials to Support Approval of Human Drugs and Biological Products" (FDA 2012), enrichment is defined as the prospective use of any patient characteristic to select a study population in which detection of an intervention effect (if one is in fact present) is more likely than it would be in an unselected population. Enrichment design is not a new idea. For example, adaptive randomization such as the play-the-winner rule with a goal to allocate more participants to the better treatment in course has been around since 1969 (Zelen 1969).

Advantages of enrichment designs include: increasing the chance of success often with a smaller sample size, directing treatment where it is likely to work best, and avoiding harm.

There are generally two kinds of enrichment, i.e., prognostic and predictive:

Prognostic Enrichment: consists of selecting participants for a trial with personal characteristics related to the disease. For example, a study of a lipid-lowering drug intended to decrease the rate of heart attacks might choose a population likely to have an increased risk of heart attacks, such as diabetics. Choosing such participants may make it more likely to observe an effect if one exists.

Predictive Enrichment: consists of applying a systematic, prespecified procedure to identify and validate a subgroup whose participants that would significantly benefit or avoid toxicity from the new therapy.

However, enrichment raises several challenging questions including (FDA 2012):

- How will data on the marker status of potential trial enrollees be used in trial design?
- How much data are needed on the unselected population?
- What types of retrospective subgroup analyses are valid (e.g., what can be reliably learned from subgroup analyses that were not prespecified in the original trial design)?

Subgroup analysis is common in clinical trials. However, the quality and level of evidence as well as the strength of conclusions regarding a subgroup-specific intervention depends on many factors including the trial design and conduct, and the reliability and predictive ability of the biomarker that defines the subgroup. Wang and Hung (2014) provide a list of criteria for consideration that may affect inter-pretability of a subgroup-specific finding. If participants with and without an enrichment characteristic are studied, then the primary result may be driven by the result in the enriched subgroup. In some enrichment designs that recruit participants with and without the enrichment characteristic, the trial-wise Type I error rate can be shared between a test conducted using only the enriched subgroup and a test conducted using the entire population. The Type I error allocation scheme allows for the assessment of the intervention effect in the entire entered population when there may be some effect in the non-enriched subgroup while also allowing assessment in the enriched subgroup. Determining the required sample size that will provide reasonable power to test these hypotheses while controlling the Type I error including a prespecified order of testing or a multiple testing procedure is challenging. Statistical methods have been discussed (e.g., Song and Chi 2007; Wang et al. 2007; Alosh and Huque 2009; Brannath et al. 2009; Mandrekar and Sargent 2009a, b; Jenkins et al. 2011; Friede et al. 2012; Millen et al. 2012; Freidlin et al. 2013; Magnusson and Turnbull 2013; Stallard et al. 2014; Graf et al. 2015). Recent developments in the statistical literature regarding identification and confirmation of targeted subgroups can be found in the *Journal of Biopharmaceutiscal Statistics* Special Issue, "Subgroup Analysis in Clinical Trials" (2014). In addition, Ondra et al. (2015) provide a systematic review on this topic.

References

Alosh M, Huque M (2009) A flexible strategy for testing subgroups and overall populations. Stat Med 28:2–23

Brannath W, Zuber E, Branson M, Bretz F, Gallo P, Posch M, Racine-Poon A (2009) Confirmatory adaptive designs with bayesian decision tools for a targeted therapy in oncology. Stat Med 28:1445–1463

Evans SR (2007) When and how can endpoints be changed after initiation of a randomized clinical trial? PLoS Clin Trials 2:e18

Evans SR, Li L, Wei LJ (2007) Data monitoring in clinical trials using prediction. Drug Inf J 41:733–742

Fine JP, Jiang H, Chappell R (2001) On semi-competing risks data. Biometrika 88:907–919

Follmann DA, Proschan MA, Geller NL (1994) Monitoring pairwise comparisons in multi-armed clinical trials. Biometrics 50:226–325

Food and Drug Administration (2012) Guidance for industry: enrichment strategies for clinical trials to support approval of human drugs and biological products. U.S. Department of Health and Human Services Food and Drug Administration, Rockville, MD, USA. Available at: http://www.fda.gov/ucm/groups/fdagov-public/@fdagov-drugs-gen/documents/document/ucm332181.pdf. Accessed 25 Nov 2015

Freidlin B, McShane LM, Korn EL (2013) Randomized clinical trials with biomarkers: design issues. J Natl Cancer Inst 102:152–160

Friede T, Parsons N, Stallard N (2012) A conditional error function approach for subgroup selection in adaptive clinical trials. Stat Med 31:4309–4320

Graf AC, Posch M, König F (2015) Adaptive designs for subpopulation analysis optimizing utility functions. Biometrical J 57:76–89

Hamasaki T, Sugimoto T, Evans SR, Sozu T (2013) Sample size determination for clinical trials with co-primary outcomes: exponential event times. Pharm Stat 12:28–34

Hung HMJ, Wang SJ, Yang P, Jin K, Lawrence J, Kordzakhia G, Massie T (2015) Statistical challenges in regulatory review of cardiovascular and CNS clinical trials. J Biopharm Stat (First published online on 14 Sept 2015 as doi:10.1080/10543406.2015.1092025)

International Conference on Harmonisation of Technical Requirements for Registration of Pharmaceuticals for Human Use (ICH) (1998) ICH harmonised tripartite guideline E9: statistical principles for clinical trials. February 1998. Available at: http://www.ich.org/fileadmin/Public_Web_Site/ICH_Products/Guidelines/Efficacy/E9/Step4/E9_Guideline.pdf. Accessed 25 Nov 2015

Jenkins M, Stone A, Jennison C (2011) An adaptive seamless phase II/III design for oncology trials with subpopulation selection using correlated survival endpoints. Pharm Stat 10:347–356

König F, Brannath W, Bretz F, Posch M (2008) Adaptive Dunnett tests for treatment selection. Stat Med 27:1612–1625

Li L, Evans SR, Uno H, Wei LJ (2009) Predicted interval plots: a graphical tool for data monitoring in clinical trials. Stat Biopharm Res 1:348–355

Magirr D, Jaki T, Whitehead J (2012) A generalized Dunnett test for multi-arm multi-stage clinical studies with treatment selection. Biometrika 99:494–501

Magnusson BP, Turnbull BW (2013) Group sequential enrichment design incorporating subgroup selection. Stat Med 32:2695–2714

Mandrekar SJ, Sargent DJ (2009a) Clinical trial designs for predictive biomarker validation: one size does not fit all. J Biopharm Stat 19:530–542

Mandrekar SJ, Sargent DJ (2009b) Clinical trial designs for predictive biomarker validation: theoretical considerations and practical challenges. J Clin Oncol 27:4027–4034

Millen BA, Dmitrienko A, Ruberg S, Shen L (2012) A statistical framework for decision making in confirmatory multipopulation tailoring clinical trials. Drug Inf J 46:647–656

Ondra T, Dmitrienko A, Friede T, Graf A, Miller F, Stallard N, Posch M (2015) Methods for identification and confirmation of targeted subgroups in clinical trials: a systematic review. J Biopharm Stat (First published online on 17 Sept 2015 as doi:10.1080/10543406.2015.1092034)

Song Y, Chi GYH (2007) A method for testing a prespecified subgroup in clinical trials. Stat Med 26:3535–3549

Stallard N, Todd S (2003) Sequential designs for phase III clinical trials incorporating treatment selection. Stat Med 22:689–703

Stallard N, Todd S (2008) A group-sequential design for clinical trials with treatment selection. Stat Med 27:6209–6227

Stallard N, Hamborg N, Parsons N, Friede T (2014) Adaptive designs for confirmatory clinical trials with subgroup selection. J Biopharm Stat 24:168–187

Sugimoto T, Sozu T, Hamasaki T, Evans SR (2013) A logrank test-based method for sizing clinical trials with two co-primary time-to-event endpoints. Biostatistics 14:409–421

Thall PF, Simon R, Ellenberg SS (1989) A two-stage design for choosing among several experimental treatments and a control in clinical trial. Biometrics 45:537–547

Wang SJ, Hung HMJ (2014) A regulatory perspective on essential considerations in design and analysis of subgroups when correctly classified. J Biopharm Stat 24:19–41

Wang SJ, O'Neill RT, Hung HMJ (2007) Approaches to evaluation of treatment effect in randomized clinical trials with genomic subset. Pharm Stat 6:244–277

Zelen M (1969) Play the winner rule and the controlled clinical trial. J Am Stat Assoc 64:131–146

Appendix A
Calculation of Power and Conditional Power in Group-Sequential Clinical Trials with Two Co-primary Endpoints

A.1 Power

The power based on DF-A discussed in Chap. 2 can be calculated by the two L-variate normal integrals and $2L$-variate normal integral are as follows:

$$1 - \beta = \Pr\left[\left\{\bigcup_{l=1}^{L} A_{1l}\right\} \cap \left\{\bigcup_{l=1}^{L} A_{2l}\right\} \middle| H_1\right]$$

$$= 1 - \left(\Pr\left[\bigcap_{l=1}^{L} D_{1l} \middle| H_0\right] + \Pr\left[\bigcap_{l=1}^{L} D_{2l} \middle| H_0\right] - \Pr\left[\bigcap_{l=1}^{L} \{D_{1l} \cap D_{2l}\} \middle| H_1\right]\right),$$

where $A_{kl} = \{Z_{kl} > c_{kl}^{E}\}$ and $D_{kl} = \{Z_{kl} \le c_{kl}^{E}\}$ ($k = 1, 2$; $l = 1, \ldots, L$).

The power based on DF-B discussed in Chap. 2 can be calculated by partitioning the set in (2.2) into mutually exclusive subsets and taking the sum of their probabilities as follows:

$$1 - \beta = \Pr\left[\bigcup_{l=1}^{L} \{A_{1l} \cap A_{2l}\} \middle| H_1\right]$$

$$= \Pr[A_{11} \cap A_{21}|H_1] + \sum_{l=2}^{L} \Pr\left[\bigcap_{l'=1}^{l-1} \{\{D_{1l'} \cup D_{2l'}\} \cap \{A_{1l} \cap A_{2l}\}\} \middle| H_1\right].$$

The probability of $\{D_{1l'} \cup D_{2l'}\}$ ($l' = 1, \ldots, l-1$) can be written as

$$\Pr[D_{1l'} \cup D_{2l'}] = \Pr[D_{1l'} \cap A_{2l'}] + \Pr[A_{1l'} \cap D_{2l'}] + \Pr[D_{1l'} \cap D_{2l'}].$$

Similarly, the probability of the union of $\{D_{1l'} \cup D_{2l'}\}$ can be written by the sum of the probabilities of the unions composed of $\{D_{1l'} \cap A_{2l'}\}$, $\{A_{1l'} \cap D_{2l'}\}$, and $\{D_{1l'} \cap D_{2l'}\}$. Then, the second term of the right-hand side in above the power can be written by

T. Hamasaki et al., *Group-Sequential Clinical Trials with Multiple Co-Objectives*, JSS Research Series in Statistics, DOI 10.1007/978-4-431-55900-9

$$\sum_{l=2}^{L} \Pr\left[\bigcap_{l'=1}^{l-1}\{\{D_{1l'} \cup D_{2l'}\} \cap \{A_{1l} \cap A_{2l}\}\}\Big|H_1\right]$$

$$= \sum_{l=2}^{L} \left(\sum_{h_l=1}^{3} \cdots \sum_{h_{l-1}=1}^{3} \Pr\left[\left\{\bigcap_{l'=1}^{l-1}\tilde{A}_{l'}^{h_{l'}}\right\} \cap \{A_{1l} \cap A_{2l}\}\Big|H_1\right]\right).$$

The probability of $\tilde{A}_{l'}^1$ is calculated by a bivariate normal integral as follows:

$$\Pr\left[\tilde{A}_{l'}^1\right] = \int_{-\infty}^{c_{1l'}} \int_{c_{2l'}}^{\infty} f_2(z_{1l'}, z_{2l'}) dz_{2l'} dz_{1l'}$$

where $f_2(z_{1l'}, z_{2l'})$ is the density function of the joint distribution of $(Z_{1l'}, Z_{2l'})$ with the means and the covariance matrix given in Sect. 2.2. The probabilities of $\tilde{A}_{l'}^2$, $\tilde{A}_{l'}^3$ and $\{A_{1l'} \cap A_{2l'}\}$ are calculated similarly. Then, the probability of the union composed of $\tilde{A}_{l'}^1$, $\tilde{A}_{l'}^2$, $\tilde{A}_{l'}^3$, and $\{A_{1l'} \cap A_{2l'}\}$ is calculated by a multivariate normal integral, and the power is the sum of $(3^L - 1)/2$ multivariate normal integrals.

For illustration, we provide the case of $L = 2$ based on DF-B. In this case, the power can be rewritten as

$$1 - \beta = \Pr[A_{1l} \cap A_{2l}|H_1] + \sum_{h_1=1}^{3} \Pr\left[\tilde{A}_1^{h_1} \cap \{A_{12} \cap A_{22}\}\Big|H_1\right]$$

$$= \int_{c_{11}}^{\infty} \int_{c_{21}}^{\infty} f_2(z_{11}, z_{21}) dz_{21} dz_{11}$$

$$+ \int_{-\infty}^{c_{11}} \int_{c_{21}}^{\infty} \int_{c_{12}}^{\infty} \int_{c_{22}}^{\infty} f_4(z_{11}, z_{21}, z_{12}, z_{22}) dz_{22} dz_{12} dz_{21} dz_{11}$$

$$+ \int_{c_{11}}^{\infty} \int_{-\infty}^{c_{21}} \int_{c_{12}}^{\infty} \int_{c_{22}}^{\infty} f_4(z_{11}, z_{21}, z_{12}, z_{22}) dz_{22} dz_{12} dz_{21} dz_{11}$$

$$+ \int_{-\infty}^{c_{11}} \int_{-\infty}^{c_{21}} \int_{c_{12}}^{\infty} \int_{c_{22}}^{\infty} f_4(z_{11}, z_{21}, z_{12}, z_{22}) dz_{22} dz_{12} dz_{21} dz_{11}$$

where $f_2(z_{11}, z_{21})$ is the density function of the bivariate normal distribution of $Z_2 = (Z_{11}, Z_{21})^T$, which is given by

$$f_2(\mathbf{Z}_2) = \frac{1}{2\pi |\mathbf{\Sigma}_2|^{1/2}} \exp\left[-\frac{1}{2}(\mathbf{Z}_2 - \boldsymbol{\mu}_2)^T \mathbf{\Sigma}_2^{-1}(\mathbf{Z}_2 - \boldsymbol{\mu}_2)\right], \quad -\infty < z_{11}, z_{21} < \infty$$

with mean vector $\boldsymbol{\mu}_2 = \sqrt{rn_1/(1+r)}(\delta_1, \delta_2)^T$ and correlation matrix

$$\mathbf{\Sigma}_2 = \begin{pmatrix} 1^2 & \rho_Z \\ \rho_Z & 1^2 \end{pmatrix}$$

where $\delta_k = (\mu_{Tk} - \mu_{Ck})/\sigma_k$ and $\rho_Z = (r\rho_T + \rho_C)/(1+r)$. In addition, $f_4(z_{11}, z_{21}, z_{12}, z_{22})$ is the density function of the tetravariate normal distribution of $Z_4 = (Z_{11}, Z_{21}, Z_{12}, Z_{22})^T$ given by

$$f_4(\mathbf{Z}_4) = \frac{1}{(2\pi)^2 |\mathbf{\Sigma}_4|^{1/2}} \exp\left[-\frac{1}{2}(\mathbf{Z}_4 - \boldsymbol{\mu}_4)^T \mathbf{\Sigma}_4^{-1}(\mathbf{Z}_4 - \boldsymbol{\mu}_4)\right], \quad -\infty < z_{11}, z_{21}, z_{12} z_{22} < \infty,$$

with mean vector $\boldsymbol{\mu}_4 = \sqrt{r/(1+r)}(\sqrt{n_1}\delta_1, \sqrt{n_1}\delta_2, \sqrt{n_2}\delta_1, \sqrt{n_2}\delta_2)^T$ and correlation matrix

$$\mathbf{\Sigma}_4 = \begin{pmatrix} \mathbf{\Sigma}_2 & \sqrt{n_1/n_2}\mathbf{\Sigma}_2 \\ \sqrt{n_1/n_2}\mathbf{\Sigma}_2 & \mathbf{\Sigma}_2 \end{pmatrix},$$

where $\mathbf{\Sigma}_4$ is positive definite matrix under $|\rho_T| < 1$ and $|\rho_C| < 1$ and $n_1 \neq n_2$ as $\mathbf{\Sigma}_4 = |\mathbf{\Sigma}_2|^2 (1 - n_1/n_2)^2$.

For details of the computation related to multivariate normal, please see Genz and Bretz (2009).

A.2 Conditional Power

The conditional power (CP) based on DF-A in Chap. 3 is

$$CP = \begin{cases} \Pr\left[\bigcup\limits_{m=S+1}^{L} A_{1m} | a_{1S}, a_{2l'}\right] \\ \quad \text{if } Z_{1l} \leq c_{1l}^E \text{ for all } l = 1, \ldots, S \text{ and } Z_{2l'} > c_{2l'}^E \text{ for some } l' = 1, \ldots, S \\ \Pr\left[\bigcup\limits_{m=S+1}^{L} A_{2m} | a_{2S}, a_{1l'}\right] \\ \quad \text{if } Z_{2l} \leq c_{2l}^E \text{ for all } l = 1, \ldots, S \text{ and } Z_{1l'} > c_{2l'}^E \text{ for some } l' = 1, \ldots, S \\ \Pr\left[\left\{\bigcup\limits_{m=S+1}^{L} A_{1m}\right\} \cap \left\{\bigcup\limits_{m=S+1}^{L} A_{2m}\right\} | a_{1S}, a_{2S}\right] \\ \quad \text{if } Z_{1l} \leq c_{1l}^E \text{ and } Z_{2l} \leq c_{2l}^E \text{ for all } l = 1, \ldots, S \end{cases}$$

where $A_{km} = \{Z_{km} > c_{km}^E\}$ and $D_{km} = \{Z_{km} \leq c_{km}^E\}$ ($k = 1, 2$; $m = S+1, \ldots, L$), and (a_{1S}, a_{2S}) is a given observed value of (Z_{1S}, Z_{2S}). The conditional distribution of $(Z_{1S+1}, \ldots, Z_{1L}, Z_{2S+1}, \ldots, Z_{2L} | a_{1S}, a_{2S})$ is a multivariate normal with means $E[Z_{km} | a_{1S}, a_{2S}] = \sqrt{n_m/2}\delta_k + \sqrt{n_S/n_m}\left(a_{kS} - \sqrt{n_m/2}\delta_k\right)$ and covariances given by $\mathrm{cov}[Z_{km}, Z_{k'm'} | a_{1S}, a_{2S}] = (n_{m'} - n_S)/\sqrt{n_m n_{m'}}$ if $k = k'$; $(n_{m'} - n_S)\rho_Z/\sqrt{n_m n_{m'}}$ if $k \neq k'$, where $m' \leq m = S+1, \ldots, L$. On the other hand, the CP based on DF-B is described by

$$\mathrm{CP} = \Pr\left[\bigcup_{m=S+1}^{L} \{A_{1m} \cap A_{2m}\} \,\middle|\, a_{1S}, a_{2S}\right] = \Pr\left[A_{1,S+1} \cap A_{2,S+1} \,\middle|\, a_{1S}, a_{2S}\right]$$

$$+ \sum_{m=S+2}^{L} \Pr\left[\bigcap_{m'=S+1}^{m-1} \{D_{1m'} \cup D_{2m'}\} \cap \{A_{1m} \cap A_{2m}\} \,\middle|\, a_{1S}, a_{2S}\right],$$

if $Z_{1l} \leq c_{1l}$ or $Z_{2l} \leq c_{2l}$ for all $l = 1, \ldots, S$. Both CP can be calculated similarly as discussed in Appendix A.

When $S = L - 1$, the CP based on DF-A can be rewritten as

$$\mathrm{CP} = \begin{cases} \Pr[A_{1L} | a_{1S}, a_{2l'}] = 1 - \Phi(c_1^*) \\ \quad \text{if } Z_{1l} \leq c_{1l}^E \text{ for all } l = 1, \ldots, S \\ \quad \text{and } Z_{2l'} > c_{2l'}^E \text{ for some } l' = 1, \ldots, S \\ \Pr[A_{2L} | a_{2S}, a_{1l'}] = 1 - \Phi(c_2^*) \\ \quad \text{if } Z_{2l} \leq c_{2l}^E \text{ for all } l = 1, \ldots, S \\ \quad \text{and } Z_{1l'} > c_{1l'}^E \text{ for some } l' = 1, \ldots, S \\ \Pr[A_{1L} \cap A_{1L} | a_{1S}, a_{2S}] = \Phi_2(-c_1^*, -c_2^* | \rho_Z) \\ \quad \text{if } Z_{1l} \leq c_{1l}^E \text{ and } Z_{2l} \leq c_{2l}^E \text{ for all } l = 1, \ldots, S \end{cases}$$

where $\Phi(\cdot)$ is the cumulative distribution function (CDF) of the standardized normal distribution and $\Phi_2(\cdot, \cdot : \rho_Z)$ is the CDF of the standard bivariate normal distribution with the correlation ρ_Z, and

$$c_k^* = \left(c_{kL}^E - a_{kS}\sqrt{n_S/n_L}\right)/\sqrt{1 - n_S/n_L} - \delta_k\sqrt{n_L - n_S}/\sqrt{2} \quad (k = 1, 2)$$

For DF-A, the CP based on DF-B can be rewritten as

$$\mathrm{CP} = \Pr[A_{1L} \cap A_{2L} | a_{1S}, a_{2S}] = \Phi_2(-c_1^*, -c_2^* | \rho_Z).$$

Genz A, Bretz F (2009) Computation of multivariate normal and t probabilities. Springer, New York

Appendix B
Efficacy and Futility Critical Boundaries and Sample Size Calculation in Group-Sequential Clinical Trials with Two Co-primary Endpoints

The efficacy and futility critical boundaries $c_{kl_k}^{\mathrm{E}}$ and $c_{kl_k}^{\mathrm{F}}$ are determined using the error-spending method to spend the Type I and Type II error rates simultaneously. $c_{kl_k}^{\mathrm{E}}$ is separately calculated for each endpoint and treated as if the endpoints are not correlated. But $c_{kl_k}^{\mathrm{F}}$ is iteratively determined by incorporating the correlations among the endpoints into the calculation with the restriction $c_{kL_k}^{\mathrm{F}} = c_{kL_k}^{\mathrm{E}}$. Here, we describe the iterative procedure to identify the efficacy and futility critical boundaries $c_{kl_k}^{\mathrm{E}}$ and $c_{kl_k}^{\mathrm{F}}$ including the calculation for MSS n_L. As a general case, we only describe the procedure based on DF-A.

Step 1: Determine $c_{k1}^{\mathrm{E}}, \ldots, c_{kL_k}^{\mathrm{E}}$ using any group-sequential method.

Step 2: Select the two initial values for MSS $n_L^{(m-1)}$ and $n_L^{(m)}$ $(m = 1, 2, \ldots)$.

Step 3: Select the initial values $\beta_k^{(j-1,m)}$ and $\beta_k^{(j,m)}$, where $\beta_k^{(j,m)}$ is the marginal Type II error rate for endpoint k $(j = 1, 2, \ldots)$.

Step 4: Calculate $n_L\left(\beta_k^{(j,m)}\right)$ and $c_{k1}^{\mathrm{F}}, \ldots, c_{kL_k}^{\mathrm{F}}$, satisfying

$$\beta_{k1}^{(j,m)} = \Pr\left[Z_{k1} \leq c_{k1}^{\mathrm{F}} | \mathrm{H}_1\right] \text{ and}$$

$$\beta_{kl}^{(j,m)} = \Pr\left[\bigcap_{l'=1}^{l-1}\{c_{kl'}^{\mathrm{F}} < Z_{kl'} \leq c_{kl'}^{\mathrm{E}}\} \cap \{Z_{kl} \leq c_{kl}^{\mathrm{F}}\} | \mathrm{H}_1\right]$$

with $\sum_{l=1}^{L_k} \beta_{kl}^{(j,m)} = \beta_k^{(j,m)}$ and $c_{kL_k}^{\mathrm{F}} = c_{kL_k}^{\mathrm{E}}$, using any group-sequential method $(k = 1, \ldots, K; l = 2, \ldots, L_k)$.

Step 5: Update the value of β_k using the equation based on basic linear interpolation

$$\beta_k^{(j+1,m)} = \frac{\beta_k^{(j-1,m)}\left\{n_L(\beta_k^{(j,m)}) - n_L^{(m)}\right\} - \beta_k^{(j,m)}\left\{n_L(\beta_k^{(j-1,m)}) - n_L^{(m)}\right\}}{n_L(\beta_k^{(j,m)}) - n_L(\beta_k^{(j-1,m)})}.$$

© The Author(s) 2016
T. Hamasaki et al., *Group-Sequential Clinical Trials with Multiple Co-Objectives*,
JSS Research Series in Statistics, DOI 10.1007/978-4-431-55900-9

Step 6: Calculate $n_L\left(\beta_k^{(j+1,m)}\right)$ and $c_{k1}^{\mathrm{F}}, \ldots, c_{kL_k}^{\mathrm{F}}$ under current $\beta_k^{(j+1,m)}$ as with Step 4.

Step 7: If $\left|\beta_k^{(j+1,m)} - \beta_k^{(j,m)}\right|$ is within a prespecified error tolerance, then stop iterative procedures with $\beta_k^{(m)}$. Otherwise, go back to Step 5. Note: Calculate $\beta_k^{(m)}$, satisfying $n_L\left(\beta_k^{(m)}\right) = n_L^{(m)}$, for all k.

Step 8: Calculate $f\left(n_L^{(m)}\right)$ which is the power (4.1) in Chap. 4 (DF-A) under the current $n_L^{(m)}$, using the $c_{k1}^{\mathrm{F}}, \ldots, c_{kL_k}^{\mathrm{F}}$ calculated at Step 6.

Step 9: Update the value of n_L, using the equation based on basic linear interpolation

$$n_L = \frac{n_L^{(m-1)}\left\{f\left(n_L^{(m)}\right) - (1-\beta)\right\} - n_L^{(m)}\left\{f\left(n_L^{(m-1)}\right) - (1-\beta)\right\}}{f\left(n_L^{(m)}\right) - f\left(n_L^{(m-1)}\right)}.$$

Step 10: If n_L is an integer, $n_L^{(m+1)} = n_L$; otherwise, $n_L^{(m+1)} = [n_L] + 1$, where $[n_L]$ is the greatest integer less than n_L. If $n_L^{(m+1)} = n_L^{(m)}$, stop the iterative procedure with $n_L^{(m+1)}$ as the final value. Otherwise, repeat Step 3–9.

Options for the two initial values $n_L^{(0)}$ and $n_L^{(1)}$ include the sample sizes calculated for detecting the smallest standardized mean differences $\min[\Delta_1, \Delta_2]$ with the marginal power $1 - \beta$ with a one-sided test at the significance level of α. Another option is calculated by the same method but with the marginal power $(1 - \beta)^{1/2}$. This is because n_L lies between these options. If all of the correlations among the endpoints are assumed to be zero, i.e., $\rho_{\mathrm{T}} = \rho_{\mathrm{C}} = 0$, and the standardized mean differences are equal, then the futility critical boundary can be simply determined, using a group-sequential method with the adjusted Type II error rate of $1 - (1 - \beta)^{1/2}$, analogous to the single primary endpoint case. However, if the endpoints are assumed to be correlated perfectly, i.e., $\rho_{\mathrm{T}} = \rho_{\mathrm{C}} = 1$, and the standardized mean differences are equal, then the futility critical boundary can be given by using a group-sequential method with the unadjusted Type II error rate of β, analogous to the single primary endpoint case. Further numerical evaluation of the behavior of the futility critical boundary will be found in Asakura et al. (2015).

Asakura K, Hamasaki T, Evans SR (2015) Interim evaluation of efficacy or futility in group-sequential clinical trials with multiple co-primary endpoints. The 2015 joint statistical meetings, Seattle, USA, August 8–13

Appendix C
ASN Calculations in Group-Sequential Clinical Trials Including Efficacy and Futility Assessments

As defined in Chap. 4, the ASN is the expected sample size under hypothetical reference values, which is given by

$$\text{ASN} = \sum_{l=1}^{L-1} n_l P_l(\delta_1, \delta_2, \sigma_1, \sigma_2, \rho_T, \rho_C)$$

$$+ n_L \left(1 - \sum_{l=1}^{L-1} n_l P_l(\delta_1, \delta_2, \sigma_1, \sigma_2, \rho_T, \rho_C) \right)$$

where $P_l(\delta_1, \delta_2, \sigma_1, \sigma_2, \rho_T, \rho_C)(=P_l) = P_l^{\text{E}} + P_l^{\text{F}}$, and P_l^{E} and P_l^{F} are the stopping probabilities as defined the likelihood of crossing the critical boundaries at the lth interim analysis assuming that the true values of the intervention's effect are (δ_1, δ_2). The ASN provides information regarding the number of participants anticipated in a group-sequential clinical trial in order to reach a decision point. We briefly describe each definition of the ASN corresponding to the decision-making frameworks described in Chap. 4.

For DF-A, the stopping probabilities at the first analysis are

$$P_1^{\text{E}} = \Pr \left[\bigcap_{k=1}^{2} A_{k1} \bigg| I_{k1} = I_1 \right] \text{ and } P_1^{\text{F}} = \Pr \left[\bigcup_{k=1}^{2} E_{k1} \bigg| I_{k1} = I_1 \right],$$

and the lth analysis $(l \geq 2)$,

$$P_l^{\text{E}} = \Pr \left[\bigcap_{k=1}^{2} \left\{ A_{k1} \cup \left\{ \bigcup_{l'_k=2}^{l_k} \left\{ \bigcap_{l''_k=1}^{l'_k-1} B_{kl''_k} \cap A_{kl'_k} \right\} \right\} \right\} \right] - \sum_{l'=1}^{l-1} P_{l'}^{\text{E}}$$

and

$$P_l^{\text{F}} = \Pr \left[\bigcup_{k=1}^{2} E_{k1} \cup \bigcup_{l'_k=2}^{l_k} \left\{ \bigcup_{k=1}^{2} \left\{ \bigcap_{l''_k=1}^{l'-1} D_{kl''_k} \right\} \cap \bigcup_{k=1}^{2} E_{kl'_k} \right\} \right] - \sum_{l'=1}^{l-1} P_{l'}^{\text{F}},$$

© The Author(s) 2016
T. Hamasaki et al., *Group-Sequential Clinical Trials with Multiple Co-Objectives*,
JSS Research Series in Statistics, DOI 10.1007/978-4-431-55900-9

where $\quad A_{kl_k} = \left\{ Z_{kl_k} > c^E_{kl_k} \right\}, \quad B_{kl_k} = \left\{ c^F_{kl_k} < Z_{kl_k} \le c^E_{kl_k} \right\}, \quad C_{kl_k} = \left\{ Z_{kl_k} > c^F_{kl_k} \right\},$

$D_{kl_k} = \left\{ Z_{kl_k} \le c^E_{kl_k} \right\}$, and $E_{kl_k} = \left\{ Z_{kl_k} \le c^F_{kl_k} \right\}$, and l_k is the latest analysis for endpoint k on or before the information time at the lth analysis (i.e., $I_{l_k} \le I_l$).

Similarly for DF-B, the stopping probabilities at the first analysis are

$$P^E_1 = \Pr\left[\bigcap_{k=1}^{2} A_{k1} \middle| I_{k1} = 1 \right] \quad \text{and} \quad P^F_1 = \Pr\left[\bigcap_{k=1}^{2} E_{k1} \middle| I_{k1} = I_1 \right],$$

and at the lth analysis $(l \ge 2)$,

$$P^E_l = \Pr\left[\bigcap_{k=1}^{2} A_{k1} \cup \bigcup_{l'_1, l'_2 = 2}^{l_1, l_2} \left\{ \bigcap_{k=1}^{2} \left\{ \bigcap_{l''_k = 1}^{l'_k - 1} C_{kl''_k} \cap A_{kl'_k} \right\} \right\} \right] - \sum_{l'=1}^{l-1} P^E_{l'}$$

and

$$P^F_l = \Pr\left[\bigcup_{l'_k = 1}^{l_k} \left\{ \bigcap_{l''_1, l''_2 = 1}^{l'_1, l'_2} \left\{ \bigcup_{k=1}^{2} D_{kl''_k} \right\} \cap \bigcup_{k=1}^{2} E_{kl'_k} \right\} \right] - \sum_{l'=1}^{l-1} P^F_{l'}.$$

Furthermore, for DF-C, the stopping probabilities at the first analysis are

$$P^E_1 = \Pr\left[\bigcap_{k=1}^{2} A_{k1} \right] \quad \text{and} \quad P^F_1 = \Pr\left[\bigcup_{k=1}^{2} E_{k1} \right],$$

and at the lth analysis $(l \ge 2)$,

$$P^E_l = \Pr\left[\bigcap_{l'=1}^{l-1} \left\{ \bigcap_{k=1}^{2} C_{kl'} \cap \bigcup_{k=1}^{2} D_{kl'} \right\} \cap \bigcap_{k=1}^{2} A_{kl} \right]$$

and

$$P^F_l = \Pr\left[\bigcap_{l'=1}^{l-1} \left\{ \bigcap_{k=1}^{2} C_{kl'} \cap \bigcup_{k=1}^{2} D_{kl'} \right\} \cap \bigcup_{k=1}^{2} E_{kl} \right],$$

where $A_{kl} = \{Z_{kl} > c^E_{kl}\}$, $C_{kl} = \{Z_{kl} > c^F_{kl}\}$, $D_{kl} = \{Z_{kl} \le c^E_{kl}\}$, and $E_{kl} = \{Z_{kl} \le c^F_{kl}\}$.

Appendix D
ASN Calculations in Three-Arm Group-Sequential Clinical Trials

The ASN is the expected sample size under hypothetical reference values and provides information regarding the number of participants anticipated in a group-sequential clinical trial in order to reach a decision point. We briefly describe the several definitions of the ASN corresponding to the decision-making frameworks.

When using DF-A or DF-B for the fixed margin and fraction approaches, if the P is not terminated until NI is demonstrated even when the AS is demonstrated at an interim analysis, then the ASN can be calculated by

$$\text{ASN1} = \sum_{l=1}^{L} N_l P_l(\mu_T, \mu_C, \mu_P, \omega, \sigma^2) + \left(1 - \sum_{l=1}^{L} P_l(\mu_T, \mu_C, \mu_P, \omega, \sigma^2)\right) N_L$$

$$= N_L + \sum_{l=1}^{L-1} (N_l - N_L) P_l(\mu_T, \mu_C, \mu_P, \omega, \sigma^2),$$

where $N_l (= n_{Tl} + n_{Cl} + n_{Pl})$ is the cumulative number of participants at the lth interim analysis and $P_l(\mu_T, \mu_C, \mu_P, \omega, \sigma^2)(=P_l)$ is the stopping probability at the lth interim analysis assuming that the true values of the intervention's means are (μ_T, μ_C, μ_P). If the analysis is conducted with equally spaced increments of information, then N_l can be rewritten as $(l/L)N_L$.

The stopping probability P_l based on DF-A is given by, for $l = 1$,

$$P_l = \Pr\left[A_1^{AS} \cap A_1^{NI}\right]$$

and for $l \geq 2$

$$P_l = \Pr\left[\bigcap_{s=1}^{l-1} B_s^{AS} \cap A_l^{AS} \cap A_l^{NI}\right] + \Pr\left[A_1^{AS} \cap \bigcap_{s=1}^{l-1} B_s^{NI} \cap A_l^{NI}\right]$$

$$+ \sum_{2 \leq s < l} \Pr\left[\bigcap_{m=1}^{s-1} B_m^{AS} \cap A_s^{AS} \cap \bigcap_{n=s}^{l-1} B_n^{NI} \cap A_l^{NI}\right],$$

T. Hamasaki et al., *Group-Sequential Clinical Trials with Multiple Co-Objectives*, JSS Research Series in Statistics, DOI 10.1007/978-4-431-55900-9 where $A_l^{AS} = \{Z_l^{AS} > c_l^{AS}\}$ and $A_l^{NI} = \{Z_l^{NI} > c_l^{NI}\}$, $B_l^{AS} = \{Z_l^{AS} \leq c_l^{AS}\}$ and $B_l^{NI} = \{Z_l^{NI} \leq c_l^{NI}\}$. For instance, at $L = 2$, the stopping probabilities P_1 and P_2 based on DF-A are calculated by multivariate normal integrals as follows:

$$P_1 = \Pr\left[A_1^{AS} \cap A_1^{NI}\right] = \int_{c_1^{AS}}^{\infty} \int_{c_1^{NI}}^{\infty} f_2\left(z_1^{AS}, z_1^{NI}\right) dz_1^{NI} dz_1^{AS}$$

and

$$P_2 = \Pr\left[B_1^{AS} \cap A_2^{AS} \cap A_2^{NI}\right] + \Pr\left[A_1^{AS} \cap B_1^{NI} \cap A_2^{NI}\right]$$

$$= \Pr\left[B_1^{AS} \cap B_1^{NI} \cap A_2^{AS} \cap A_2^{NI}\right] + \Pr\left[B_1^{AS} \cap A_1^{NI} \cap A_2^{AS} \cap A_2^{NI}\right]$$

$$+ \Pr\left[A_1^{AS} \cap B_1^{NI} \cap A_2^{AS} \cap A_2^{NI}\right] + \Pr\left[A_1^{AS} \cap B_1^{NI} \cap B_2^{AS} \cap A_2^{NI}\right]$$

$$= \int_{-\infty}^{c_1^{AS}} \int_{-\infty}^{c_1^{NI}} \int_{c_2^{AS}}^{\infty} \int_{c_2^{NI}}^{\infty} f_4\left(z_1^{AS}, z_1^{NI}, z_2^{AS}, z_2^{NI}\right) dz_2^{NI} dz_2^{AS} dz_1^{NI} dz_1^{AS}$$

$$+ \int_{-\infty}^{c_1^{AS}} \int_{c_1^{NI}}^{\infty} \int_{c_2^{AS}}^{\infty} \int_{c_2^{NI}}^{\infty} f_4\left(z_1^{AS}, z_1^{NI}, z_2^{AS}, z_2^{NI}\right) dz_2^{NI} dz_2^{AS} dz_1^{NI} dz_1^{AS}$$

$$+ \int_{c_1^{AS}}^{\infty} \int_{-\infty}^{c_1^{NI}} \int_{c_2^{AS}}^{\infty} \int_{c_2^{NI}}^{\infty} f_4\left(z_1^{AS}, z_1^{NI}, z_2^{AS}, z_2^{NI}\right) dz_2^{NI} dz_2^{AS} dz_1^{NI} dz_1^{AS}$$

$$+ \int_{c_1^{AS}}^{\infty} \int_{-\infty}^{c_1^{NI}} \int_{-\infty}^{c_2^{AS}} \int_{c_2^{NI}}^{\infty} f_4\left(z_1^{AS}, z_1^{NI}, z_2^{AS}, z_2^{NI}\right) dz_2^{NI} dz_2^{AS} dz_1^{NI} dz_1^{AS}$$

where $f_l(\cdot)$ is the probability density function of l multivariate normal distribution under the alternative hypotheses H_1^{AS} and H_1^{NI}. On the other hand, the stopping probability P_l based on DF-B is given by, for $l = 1$,

$$P_l = \Pr\left[A_1^{AS} \cap A_1^{NI}\right],$$

and, for $l \geq 2$,

$$P_l = \Pr\left[\bigcap_{s=1}^{l-1} \{B_s^{AS} \cup B_s^{NI}\} \cap A_l^{AS} \cap A_l^{NI}\right].$$

When using DF-A for the fixed margin approach, we have an option for discontinuing the placebo group at the interim when the AS is demonstrated. In this situation, the ASN can be calculated by

$$
\text{ASN2} = \sum_{l=1}^{L} \sum_{s=1}^{l} \{N_l - (n_{Pl} - n_{Ps})\} P_{l|s}\left(\mu_T, \mu_C, \mu_P, \omega, \sigma^2\right) + \left(1 - \sum_{l=1}^{L} P_l\right) N_L
$$

$$
= N_L + \sum_{l=1}^{L} \sum_{s=1}^{l} \{N_l - N_L - (n_{Pl} - n_{Ps})\} P_{l|s}\left(\mu_T, \mu_C, \mu_P, \omega, \sigma^2\right),
$$

where $P_{l|s}(\mu_T, \mu_C, \mu_P, \omega, \sigma^2) = P_{l|s}$ is given by

$$
P_{l|s} = \begin{cases}
\Pr\left[A_1^{AS} \cap A_1^{NI}\right], & \text{if } l = s = 1, \\[2ex]
\Pr\left[\bigcap_{s=1}^{l-1} B_s^{AS} \cap A_l^{AS} \cap A_l^{NI}\right], & \text{if } l = s \geq 2, \\[2ex]
\Pr\left[A_1^{AS} \cap \bigcap_{s=1}^{k-1} B_s^{NI} \cap A_l^{NI}\right], & \text{if } l > s = 1, \\[2ex]
\Pr\left[\bigcap_{m=1}^{s-1} B_m^{AS} \cap A_s^{AS} \cap \bigcap_{n=s}^{l-1} B_n^{NI} \cap A_l^{NI}\right], & \text{if } l > s \geq 2.
\end{cases}
$$

Printed in the United States
By Bookmasters